Updates in Surgery

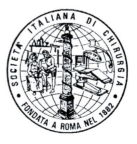

Lorenzo Capussotti (Ed.)

Surgical Treatment of Colorectal Liver Metastases

In collaboration with
Alessandro Ferrero
Andrea Muratore
Dario Ribero
Luca Viganò

Forewords by
Enrico De Antoni
Gennaro Nuzzo

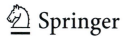

Editor
Lorenzo Capussotti
Chief of the Surgical Department
Director of the Division of Hepato-Bilio-Pancreatic and Digestive Surgery
Mauriziano "Umberto I" Hospital
Turin, Italy

In collaboration with
Alessandro Ferrero
Andrea Muratore
Dario Ribero
Luca Viganò
Division of Hepato-Bilio-Pancreatic and Digestive Surgery
Mauriziano "Umberto I" Hospital
Turin, Italy

The publication and the distribution of this volume have been supported by the Italian Society of Surgery

ISBN 978-88-470-1808-2   e-ISBN 978-88-470-1809-9

DOI 10.1007/978-88-470-1809-9

Springer Milan Dordrecht Heidelberg London New York

Library of Congress Control Number: 2010933718

© Springer-Verlag Italia 2011

This work is subject to copyright. All rights are reserved, whether the whole or part of the material is concerned, specifically the rights of translation, reprinting, reuse of illustrations, recitation, broadcasting, reproduction on microfilm or in any other way, and storage in data banks. Duplication of this publication or parts thereof is permitted only under the provisions of the Italian Copyright Law in its current version, and permission for use must always be obtained from Springer. Violations are liable to prosecution under the Italian Copyright Law.

The use of general descriptive names, registered names, trademarks, etc. in this publication does not imply, even in the absence of a specific statement, that such names are exempt from the relevant protective laws and regulations and therefore free for general use.

Product liability: The publishers cannot guarantee the accuracy of any information about dosage and application contained in this book. In every individual case the user must check such information by consulting the relevant literature.

Cover design: Simona Colombo, Milan, Italy
Typesetting: Graphostudio, Milan, Italy
Printing and binding: Arti Grafiche Nidasio, Assago (MI), Italy

Printed in Italy

Springer-Verlag Italia S.r.l. – Via Decembrio 28 – I-20137 Milan
Springer is a part of Springer Science+Business Media (www.springer.com)

Foreword

The management of colorectal liver metastases is one of the most rapidly changing areas in medicine. Over the last few decades, diagnostic imaging has tremendously improved, surgical indications and techniques have rapidly evolved, and newer and effective chemotherapies have expanded the armamentarium of medical oncologists. These achievements have, in turn, compelled physicians to redefine existing treatment strategies in recognition of the possibility of cure in patients who just a few years ago were deemed to have incurable disease. The restless work of innovative surgeons has established the value of an aggressive surgical attitude and has brought about a profound revision of long-standing criteria of resectability. New techniques have been developed, overcoming many of the previous limits of surgery. Similarly, chemotherapy is no longer considered only for palliative treatments but is now an essential adjunct to surgery in a modern multidisciplinary approach. *Surgical Treatment of Colorectal Liver Metastases* addresses the contemporary multidisciplinary management of liver metastases. It logically and informatively provides an up-to-date, accurate summary of the indications, results, technologies, methodologies and other related issues relevant to the surgical management of colorectal metastatic disease.

It is with great pleasure and keen interest that the Italian Society of Surgery offers its members and the medical community at large the opportunity to broaden their knowledge in this particular field of surgery. We therefore highly appreciate the efforts of one of our members, Prof. Lorenzo Capussotti, of the Hepato-Bilio-Pancreatic and Digestive Surgery Department, Mauriziano "Umberto I" Hospital (Turin, Italy) for this extraordinary work. I am convinced that *Surgical Treatment of Colorectal Liver Metastases* will be enthusiastically received, based on its great scientific and practical value as an essential reference for all surgeons involved in the treatment of patients with liver metastases.

Rome, October 2010

Enrico De Antoni
President, Italian Society of Surgery

Foreword

No other branch of digestive surgery has undergone the profound changes that have taken place in hepatic surgery in recent years, especially as a result of the application of functional segmental liver anatomy and intraoperative ultrasound in resective surgery. At the same time, the extraordinary progresses achieved in medical oncology together with the close cooperation between surgeons and oncologists has led to a watershed in this field of medicine, especially with respect to colorectal liver metastases.

Hepatic surgery is therefore a topic of great interest and the Italian Society of Surgery, by assigning Lorenzo Capussotti the task of authoring the biennial report, has rightly recognized his important contributions to the current state of the art. Indeed a PubMed search will immediately show that there is no aspect of liver surgery that does not include articles published by him and his research group in major international journals with high impact factors.

Lorenzo Capussotti is one of the leading lights on the international stage of hepatic surgery. With his enthusiasm, persistence, and charisma he has formed a group in Turin that has become a point of reference in the field. Moreover, he has created an international network that has allowed Italian resective liver surgery to reach the highest summits in the world.

This biennial report covers the topic with extreme thoroughness. Diagnostics, indications, surgical techniques, surgical risks, and long-term results are discussed in great detail. The contribution of original ideas, the fruit of considerable personal experience, is invaluable, as is the discussion of their application in clinical practice. Capussotti's surgery unit is the ideal example of a surgical department oriented not only towards healthcare but also towards research.

Pervading the report is the importance of interdisciplinary cooperation, particularly with radiologists, oncologists, and pathologists. Today, such cooperation is indispensable in the surgical treatment of an increasing number of patients considered as recently as only a few years ago to have inoperable disease, and in obtaining results that previously could not be expected.

The fluency of Lorenzo Capussotti's style, his ability to summarize complex issues, and the clarity of the message he presents deserve particular mention. Not only our colleagues in the field of hepatic surgery but also those with other medical interests will find this book to be a precious source of up-to-date information and readily appreciate its value in daily practice.

The invitation I received from Lorenzo to author this Foreword was an honor and further proof of our valued friendship.

Rome, October 2010

Gennaro Nuzzo
Unit of Hepato-Biliary Surgery
Università Cattolica del Sacro Cuore
Policlinico A. Gemelli
Rome, Italy

Preface

Liver surgery is the only potentially curative treatment of colorectal liver metastases. This concept has been accepted since the beginning of the 1980s and is still absolutely valid 30 years later. Initial reluctance to surgically treat metastatic diseases has been completely overcome by the achieved survival results and the demonstrated superiority of hepatic resection to palliative treatments. No medical or alternative interventional procedure has yielded results similar to those reported after radical liver resection. Currently, radical surgery not only represents the gold standard in the treatment of colorectal liver metastases, but it is also the final aim of any medical strategy aimed at this disease.

Reported survival benefits from radical resection have encouraged a continuous extension of the surgical indications. Consequently, synchronous, multiple, bilobar, and large metastases are now currently scheduled for resection, and neither vascular or biliary infiltration nor the presence of resectable extrahepatic disease is a contraindication to resection. The only limit is the technical feasibility of complete resection. Moreover, complex surgical strategies, including induced parenchymal hypertrophy through portal vein occlusion, ultrasound-guided parenchymal sparing resections, and two-stage procedures, have been devised and are pushing the limits of this therapeutic approach. These techniques have been made possible and further enhanced by refinements in surgical technique, anesthesiologist assistance and liver anatomy and physiology knowledge. Together, they have rendered hepatic surgery a standardized and safe procedure. Mortality rates have fallen and are currently below 1–2%.

The history and evolution of surgery for colorectal liver metastases cannot ignore chemotherapy. After the introduction of oxaliplatin- and irinotecan-based regimens, chemotherapy has played an indispensable ancillary role. Hope of cure has been extended to patients with initially unresectable disease due to unexpected tumor shrinkage during chemotherapy, which has enabled secondary resection. The concept of "conversion" treatment was coined to underline this switch from a palliative to a potentially curative scenario. In patients with resectable disease, chemotherapy has improved surgical results by allowing the selection of candidates for resection and by reducing, or at least delaying, postoperative recurrences. The recent advent of biologics has further strengthened cooperation between surgical and medical approaches. Nonetheless, despite these excellent results, drawbacks associated with chemotherapy and the use of biologics have been pointed out, such that an optimal cooperation between surgery and medical treatments has yet to be found.

In the last few years, interventional procedures have complemented surgery in terms of achieving complete eradication of colorectal liver metastases. Radiofrequency thermal ablation, cryotherapy, and microwave ablation are not, per se, curative procedures and should not be considered as alternatives to resection. However, in patients facing complex surgical procedures, interstitial treatments may overcome the ill-location limits of some metastases and increase the possibility of resection in otherwise unresectable cases.

The complexity and multiplicity of the surgical approaches to colorectal liver metastases has resulted in many controversial and unresolved issues. Increasingly, however, published experiences are providing answers to the many outstanding questions. Nonetheless, evidence-based guidelines for clinical practice are lacking and their definition has been hindered by difficulties in accruing patients, inhomogeneous cohort characteristics, the rapid evolution of indications and treatment strategies, and the different policies followed in different centers. The establishment of a multicentric prospective database could solve many clinical dilemmas by collecting large number of patients. Indeed, the LiverMetSurvey registry currently represents the largest worldwide effort, having catalogued more than 10,000 cases.

The aim of the present book is to elucidate the role of surgery in the therapeutic approach to colorectal liver metastases, with special emphasis on the indications for resection, the results of this procedure, and its matters of debate. An extensive literature review provides the basis for every chapter, allowing an analysis of current levels of evidence. The different results accumulated by worldwide centers and the many different opinions concerning hepatic resection in patients with colorectal liver metastases have been integrated with those of our center. Medical treatments and interventional procedures complementary to surgery are evaluated, omitting their exclusive application in the palliative setting.

Turin, October 2010   **Lorenzo Capussotti**

Contents

1 Epidemiology and Natural History 1

    1.1   Introduction 1
    1.2   Epidemiology 2
    1.3   Natural History and Disease Therapy 4
    References 6

2 Diagnosis and Staging 7

    2.1   Introduction 7
    2.2   Ultrasonography 8
    2.3   Computed Tomography 10
    2.4   Magnetic Resonance Imaging 13
    2.5   Performance and Comparison of Imaging Modalities 16
    2.6   Positron Emission Tomography 19
    2.7   Diagnosis and Staging of Liver Metastases from Colorectal Cancer ... 22
    2.8   Liver Metastases Detection After Chemotherapy 23
    References 24

3 Evolution of Resectability Criteria 27

    3.1   Introduction 27
    3.2   Resectability Criteria 28
    3.3   Resection Margin 31
    References 32

4 Surgical Strategy 35

    4.1   Introduction 35
    4.2   Intraoperative Ultrasonography 36

4.3	Parenchyma-sparing Surgery	43
4.4	Laparoscopic Liver Resection	45
4.5	Hepatic Pedicle Clamping	48
References		50

5 Results of Surgery and Prognostic Factors ... 55

5.1	Introduction	55
5.2	Short-term Results	56
5.3	Long-term Results	58
5.4.	Prognostic Factors	61
References		71

6 Preoperative Chemotherapy ... 75

6.1	Introduction	75
6.2	Unresectable Liver Metastases	76
6.3	Resectable Liver Metastases	85
6.4	Chemotherapy-related Liver Injuries	89
6.5	Disappeared Liver Metastases	94
References		96

7 Synchronous Colorectal Liver Metastases ... 101

7.1	Introduction	101
7.2	Resectable Synchronous Liver Metastases	102
7.3	Unresectable Synchronous Liver Metastases	110
7.4	Conclusions	115
References		116

8 Therapeutic Strategies in Unresectable Colorectal Liver Metastases ... 121

8.1	Introduction	121
8.2	Portal Vein Occlusion	122
8.3	Two-stage Hepatectomy	126
8.4	Interstitial Treatments	130
References		135

9 Extrahepatic Disease ... 139

9.1	Introduction	139
9.2	Lymph-node Metastases	140
9.3	Peritoneal Carcinomatosis	143
9.4	Pulmonary Metastases	145

9.5	Other Sites		147
9.6	Conclusions		148
References			149

10 Adjuvant Chemotherapy and Follow-Up 153

10.1	Introduction		153
10.2	Adjuvant Chemotherapy		154
10.3	Follow-Up		155
References			156

11 Re-resection: Indications and Results 159

11.1	Introduction		159
11.2	Short-term Outcome		160
11.3	Long-term Outcome		161
References			162

12 LiverMetSurvey Registry: the Italian Experience 165

12.1	Introduction		165
12.2	The Italian Experience		167
12.3	Conclusions		182

Subject Index 183

Contributors

Massimo Aglietta
Medical Oncology, University of Turin
Division of Medical Oncology
Institute for Cancer Research
and Treatment
Candiolo (TO), Italy

Marco Amisano
Division of Hepato-Bilio-Pancreatic and
Digestive Surgery
Mauriziano "Umberto I" Hospital
Turin, Italy

Lorenzo Capussotti
Surgical Department
Division of Hepato-Bilio-Pancreatic and
Digestive Surgery
Mauriziano "Umberto I" Hospital
Turin, Italy

Stefano Cirillo
Radiology Unit
Mauriziano "Umberto I" Hospital
Turin, Italy

Alessandro Ferrero
Division of Hepato-Bilio-Pancreatic and
Digestive Surgery
Mauriziano "Umberto I" Hospital
Turin, Italy

Teresa Gallo
Radiology Unit
Mauriziano "Umberto I" Hospital
Turin, Italy

Serena Langella
Division of Hepato-Bilio-Pancreatic and
Digestive Surgery
Mauriziano "Umberto I" Hospital
Turin, Italy

Francesco Leone
Division of Medical Oncology
Institute for Cancer Research
and Treatment
Candiolo (TO), Italy

Roberto Lo Tesoriere
Division of Hepato-Bilio-Pancreatic and
Digestive Surgery
Mauriziano "Umberto I" Hospital
Turin, Italy

Annalisa Macera
Radiology Unit
Mauriziano "Umberto I" Hospital
Turin, Italy

Andrea Muratore
Division of Hepato-Bilio-Pancreatic and
Digestive Surgery
Mauriziano "Umberto I" Hospital
Turin, Italy

Dario Ribero
Division of Hepato-Bilio-Pancreatic and
Digestive Surgery
Mauriziano "Umberto I" Hospital
Turin, Italy

Nadia Russolillo
Division of Hepato-Bilio-Pancreatic and
Digestive Surgery
Mauriziano "Umberto I" Hospital
Turin, Italy

Elisa Sperti
Unit of Medical Oncology
Mauriziano "Umberto I" Hospital
Turin, Italy

Luca Viganò
Division of Hepato-Bilio-Pancreatic and
Digestive Surgery
Mauriziano "Umberto I" Hospital
Turin, Italy

Giuseppe Zimmitti
Division of Hepato-Bilio-Pancreatic and
Digestive Surgery
Mauriziano "Umberto I" Hospital
Turin, Italy

Epidemiology and Natural History

1

Abstract Although the vast majority of patients with a large-bowel primary have tumors amenable to curative resection at the time of diagnosis, the disease recurs in more than half of the patients, with the liver involved in up to two-thirds of the cases. Synchronous liver metastases are diagnosed in approximately 15% of the cases. In such patients, liver disease represents the sole site of distant metastases in more than 75%. Metachronous liver metastases develop in 16–20% of patients usually within the first 3 years. Untreated liver metastases have a grim prognosis. Liver resection is the only potentially curative treatment although only 20% of patients can be considered as candidates for surgery.

1.1
Introduction

Colorectal cancer is the fourth most common neoplasm worldwide, with approximately 1.2 million new cases diagnosed each year [1]. Significant international variations in the number of incident cases have been observed, with the highest rates reported in Europe, North America, and Oceania [2].

In Italy, based on data from the Italian Network of Cancer Registries (AIRTUM), which collects epidemiologic information from both general and specialized population-based cancer registries covering more than 32% of the entire Italian resident population (approximately 19,000,000 people), it has been estimated that in 2010 more than 29,200 new cases of colorectal cancers will be diagnosed among men and more than 17,500 among women. These crude numbers correspond to a cumulative risk (0–74 years) of developing a colon cancer of about 34.3‰ in men (i.e., 1 case every 29 men) and 22.2‰ in women (i.e., 1 case every 45 women) [3]. Mortality trend analyses for selected countries across the globe reporting highly accurate long-term mortality data have demonstrated that, in the period 1995–2005, colorectal cancer mortality significantly decreased in both males and females in longstanding, economically developed nations such as the United States, Australia, and the majority

D. Ribero (✉)
Division of Hepato-Bilio-Pancreatic and Digestive Surgery, Mauriziano "Umberto I" Hospital, Turin, Italy

Surgical Treatment of Colorectal Liver Metastases. Lorenzo Capussotti (Ed.)
© Springer-Verlag Italia 2011

1

of Western Europe. Nonetheless, colorectal cancer still represents the second leading cause of cancer-related deaths. In fact, even though 85% of patients with a large-bowel primary have tumors amenable to curative resection at the time of diagnosis, the disease recurs in more than half of the patients, with the liver involved in up to two-thirds of the cases.

In most of the surgical literature on colorectal liver metastases, concise epidemiologic information on the incidence of synchronous and metachronous hepatic metastases and on resectability rates are provided, usually with reference to hospital-based reports. However, these data are limited by recruitment bias, since they are extrapolated from series of patients referred to tertiary care centers. Therefore, these incidence rates cannot be regarded as reference values for the entire population. Rather, population-based studies are essential for providing non-biased, truly representative data on the incidence, management, and prognosis of hepatic synchronous and metachronous metastases. Yet, such studies are rare because of the inherent problems in data collection from the entire population of patients with large-bowel cancer within a particular area. In the following, epidemiologic data will be discussed based on the few available studies conducted at a population level [4-6].

1.2
Epidemiology

The incidence of synchronous metastases has been reported to vary widely, between 15 and 30%. Using a population-based cancer registry, Manfredi et al. [4] recently analyzed 13,463 patients diagnosed with a large-bowel cancer over a 25-year period (1976–2000) in two administrative French areas, the Côte-d'Or and the Saône-et-Loire, with a resident population of more than 1 million people. The incidence of individuals with synchronous liver metastases identified during the diagnostic workup or in the course of treatment was 14.5%. Similar data have been reported in previous studies from Western Europe [7], France [8], and Australia [9]. In approximately 77% of the cases, Manfredi et al. [4] found that liver metastases were the sole distant secondary tumor, while in 23% of the cases they were associated with other visceral metastases. Synchronous liver metastases were more frequent in males (15.9%) than in females (12.8%), with age-standardized incidence rates of 7.6 and 3.7 per 100,000, respectively (sex ratio 2.1). Interestingly, the incidence of synchronous liver metastases was significantly influenced by the age at diagnosis: 19.8% before age 55, 16.7% between 55 and 64, 16.0% between 65 and 74, and 11.7% in patients 75 and over. Conversely, no correlation was demonstrated with the site of the primary tumor: 14.8% for colon cancers and 13.9% for rectal cancer. Compared to patients who developed secondary liver tumors after the treatment of their primary tumor, patients with synchronous metastases exhibited a higher number of liver deposits and a more frequent bilobar distribution. Rather disappointingly, analysis of temporal trends showed that the incidence of synchronous liver metastases was relatively stable over time. This is probably attributable to advances in preoperative imaging coupled with the implementation of screening programs. These two factors result in an increase in the proportion of tumors discovered with synchronous metastases counterbalanced by an increase in the number of asymptomatic patients diagnosed at stage I.

In a separate study, using the Côte-d'Or cancer registry, the authors analyzed the pattern of failure after resection for cure of colonic cancer [5]. The 5-year overall incidence of tumor relapse was 31.5%. More than 12% of patients developed local recurrence, usually within the first 3 years. Cancers of the rectosigmoid junction were more prone to local recurrence than tumors of the right or left colon. Emergency surgery was also associated with increased recurrence, but there was no significant difference between operations performed for obstructing and perforated tumors. Local recurrence was associated with distant metastases in half of the patients. Distant metastases, without local recurrence were diagnosed in 23.9% of patients. Similar to local recurrence, almost 80% of distant metastases occurred within 3 years following the diagnosis of colon cancer. Metastatic disease was confined to the liver in 43.5% of the patients, the peritoneum in 14.6%, the lung in 10.2%, the brain in 1.7%, bone in 1.9%, and to other sites in 4.1%; multiple organ involvement was observed in one out of five patients. Not unexpectedly, there was a significant increase in the cumulative rate of distant metastasis with increasing penetration of the primary tumor; the 5-year cumulative risk was 6.4% for stage I, 21.4% for stage II, and 48% for stage III tumors. This means that there was a 6.1-fold increase in the relative risk of recurrence for T4 *vs.* T1 tumors and a 4.6-fold increase for N2 *vs.* N0 tumors. When the analysis was focused on the risk of developing metachronous metastases to the liver, two studies from different populations reported an overall actuarial cumulative rate of 4–4.3% at 1 year, 8.7–12% at 3 years, 13.5% at 3 years, and 16.5% at 5 years [4, 6]. In none of these studies did cancer site significantly influence the occurrence of metachronous liver metastasis, in contrast to the stage of the primary at diagnosis. In particular, there was a nearly eight-fold increase in the relative risk of liver metastasis for stage III lesions compared with stage I lesions.

Similar data were obtained in our series of 874 patients who had undergone curative intent resection of a colorectal carcinoma between January 2000 and June 2007 (unpublished data). However, in our cohort, rectal cancer patients had a higher rate of tumor relapse that was more pronounced in lower stages. In fact, the overall recurrence rate in patients with stage I and II colon cancers was 5.3% vs. 12.5% for stage I and II naïve rectal cancers and 26.3% for stage I and II rectal cancers after neoadjuvant therapy. In addition, patients with rectal cancer had a significantly higher rate of lung and local recurrences than was the case in colon cancer patients. An additional interesting finding was that the median time-to-recurrence was different according to the site of metastases, with liver recurrences appearing significantly earlier than those of the lung. Of note, the only other clinical variable influencing the time-to-recurrence was the primary tumor stage. Recurrences after resection of stage I or II cancer occurred significantly later than after resection of more advanced tumors.

1.3
Natural History and Disease Therapy

The natural history of untreated metastatic colorectal cancer is the standard against which the effectiveness of any treatment should be measured. However, since in the past 30 years most clinicians have been unwilling to leave patients with stage IV disease untreated, it is difficult to define the natural history when so little is left to nature. Using historical controls from the 1970s, authors reported that without treatment the median survival for patients with colorectal liver metastases was only 6–12 months [10, 11], varying with the extent of disease at presentation. The prognosis was somewhat better for those who had limited involvement of the liver [12]. In a 1984 study, Wagner et al. [13] reported that the median survival of patients who had unresected solitary and multiple unilobar lesions was 21 and 15 months, respectively. However, according to two studies, one in the 1970s and the other in the 1980s, even for the best prognostic groups, only 77% of patients were alive at 1 year, with only 14–23% surviving more than 3 years [13, 14]. On a population-based level, approximately 70% of the patients with untreated hepatic metastasis succumbed within 1 year and only a few (0.4–4%) survived 5 years [4, 15]. With recent substantial advances in medical and surgical oncology, the fate of patients with colorectal metastases has dramatically changed. Until 1998, when fluorouracil and leucovorin were the sole therapeutic options for patients with unresectable disease, median overall survival times were stagnant at approximately 8–12 months. In a 2009 population-based study analyzing 2470 patients from two academic centers in the United States, Kopetz et al. [16] showed that there was no significant difference in median overall survival for patients diagnosed from 1990 through 1997, while significant improvements were seen thereafter (from 18 months in 1998–2000 to 29.2 months in 2004–2006) (Fig. 1.1a). In particular, the authors demonstrated that these developments occurred in two stages. The first started with patients diagnosed in 1998 and was associated with increased utilization of hepatic resection. After an initial rapid incorporation of this surgical approach into clinical practice, the number of patients undergoing hepatic resection has since stabilized at approximately 20% (Fig. 1.1b) [16]. This proportion, as well as the temporal trend, is similar to what has been reported in other population-based studies [4, 6]. Interestingly, the authors showed that the degree of benefit from hepatic resection was tremendous. In fact, increasing hepatic resection rates from 6% to 20% of the metastatic population–still a small proportion of the entire population—provided an overall population survival benefit similar to the benefit of front-line treatment derived by the addition of irinotecan to fluorouracil in the entire population. In addition, it should be noted that these changes were almost entirely related to the increased frequency with which hepatectomies were performed for metachronous metastases. In fact, reports indicate not only that is resection for cure less often performed in synchronous metastases but also that the proportion of resected synchronous liver metastasis did not significantly increase over time [4]. The second stage of survival gains started in 2004 and is most likely attributable to medical therapy. Around this time, several additional drugs

1 Epidemiology and Natural History

became available for use in the United States, including oxaliplatin, bevacizumab, and cetuximab. Notably, improvements after 2004 have correlated with a rapid increase in the use of these agents (Fig. 1.2).

Although tumor recurrence after curative treatment of a colorectal primary still

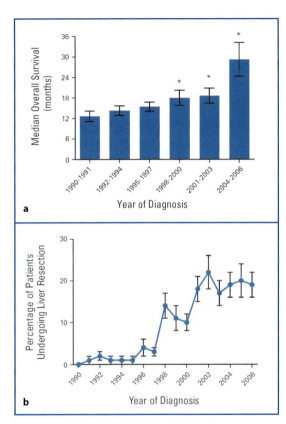

Fig. 1.1 a Median overall survival of 2470 patients with metastatic colorectal cancer treated at the M.D. Anderson Cancer Center and the Mayo Clinic, as shown by year of diagnosis. Error bars represent 95% CIs; *significant improvements vs. the preceding period. **b** The percentage of patients undergoing liver resection by date of diagnosis increased significantly for patients diagnosed in 1998 and stabilized around 20% for patients diagnosed in 2000–2006. Error bars represent SEM. (From Kopetz et al [16], reprinted with permission. © 2008 American Society of Clinical Oncology. All rights reserved)

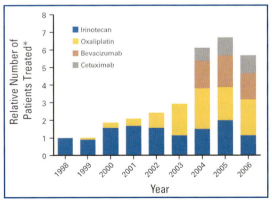

Fig. 1.2 Temporal trends in the use of various chemotherapeutics. (From Kopetz et al [16], reprinted with permission. © 2008 American Society of Clinical Oncology. All rights reserved)

represents a major problem, both the use of hepatic resection and improved chemotherapy have significantly changed the natural history of metastatic tumors in patients, providing prolonged survival and in some cases the hope for cure.

References

1. Parkin DM, Bray F, Ferlay J et al (2005) Global cancer statistics, 2002. CA Cancer J Clin 55:74–108
2. Center MM, Jemal A, Smith RA et al (2009) Worldwide variations in colorectal cancer. CA Cancer J Clin 59:366–378
3. Italian cancer trends (1998-2005). Report 2009. Available at http://www.registri-tumori.it/PDF/AIRTUM2009Trend/E&P33_4-5S1_38_colonretto.pdf. Accessed May, 15th, 2010
4. Manfredi S, Lepage C, Hatem C et al (2006) Epidemiology and management of liver metastases from colorectal cancer. Ann Surg 244:254–259
5. Manfredi S, Bouvier AM, Lepage C et al (2006) Incidence and patterns of recurrence after resection for cure of colonic cancer in a well defined population. Br J Surg 93:1115–1122
6. Leporrier J, Maurel J, Chiche L et al (2006) A population-based study of the incidence, management and prognosis of hepatic metastases from colorectal cancer. Br J Surg 93:465–474
7. Gatta G, Capocaccia R, Sant M et al (2000) Understanding variations in survival for colorectal cancer in Europe: a EUROCARE high resolution study. Gut 47:533–538
8. Phelip JM, Grosclaude P, Launoy G (2005) Are there regional differences in the management of colon cancer in France? Eur J Cancer 131:504–510
9. Kune GA, Kune S, Field B et al (1990) Survival in patients with large-bowel cancer: a population-based investigation from the Melbourne Colorectal Cancer Study. Dis Colon Rectum 33:938–946
10. Bengtsson G, Carlsson G, Hafstrom L et al (1981) Natural history of patients with untreated liver metastases from colorectal cancer. Am J Surg 141:586–589
11. Norstein J, Silen W (1997) Natural history of liver metastases from colo-rectal carcinoma. J Gastrointest Surg 1:398–407
12. Stangl R, Altendorf-Hofmann A, Charnley RM et al (1994) Factors influencing the natural history of colorectal liver metastases. Lancet 343:1405–1410
13. Wagner JS, Adson MA, Adson MH et al (1984) The natural history of hepatic metastases from colorectal cancer. A comparison with resective treatment. Ann Surg 199:502–507
14. Wood CB, Gillis CR, Blumgart LH (1976) A retrospective study of the natural history of patients with liver metastases from colorectal cancer. Clin Oncol 2:285–288
15. Rougier P, Milan C, Lazorthes F et al (1995) Prospective study of prognostic factors in patients with unresected metastases from colorectal cancer. Br J Surg 82:1397–1400
16. Kopetz S, Chang GJ, Overman MJ et al (2009) Improved survival in metastatic colorectal cancer is associated with adoption of hepatic resection and improved chemotherapy. J Clin Oncol 27:3677–3683

Diagnosis and Staging

2

Abstract Over the past several decades, the 5-year survival rates after resection of colorectal liver metastases have almost doubled, from about 30% to about 60%. Among other factors, this improved survival has been attributed to better preoperative imaging techniques, which have improved patient selection. In patients being considered for surgical therapy of hepatic colorectal metastases, a high-quality cross-sectional imaging study, either contrast-enhanced CT or MRI, should be performed to evaluate these metastases before surgery. MRI, however, is inferior to CT in the evaluation of extrahepatic disease but superior in patients after preoperative chemotherapy. PET/CT appears to improve patient selection and should be considered as part of the preoperative evaluation of resectability in high-risk patients.

2.1
Introduction

The liver is the first and most common site of metastatic spread from colorectal carcinoma. In studies reporting on autopsy results, metastases involve up to 70% of patients. Metastases are confined to the liver in 30–40% of patients at the time of detection [1, 2]. In patients with metastatic colorectal cancer, imaging plays a principal role in screening for disease presence, tumor staging, evaluation of the response to treatment, and surveillance for tumor recurrence following surgery.

The choice of the optimal treatment strategy in patients with liver metastases depends on general clinical data but is mainly based upon an accurate assessment of the imaging characteristics of both the liver and the hepatic lesions, including their number, size and location, type of tissue, and the number of involved liver segments [3]. A detailed mapping of metastatic liver involvement is therefore essential to define the most adequate and effective treatment.

Pre-operative staging is important in patient selection to avoid inappropriate surgery [4, 5]. Evaluation of tumor resectability includes assessment of vascular structures for tumor invasion and vascular anomalies. The evolution of imaging over the

S. Cirillo (✉)
Radiology Unit, Mauriziano "Umberto I" Hospital, Turin, Italy

Surgical Treatment of Colorectal Liver Metastases. Lorenzo Capussotti (Ed.)
© Springer-Verlag Italia 2011

past several decades has allowed earlier, more accurate detection and characterization of colorectal liver metastases. The current challenge for diagnostic imaging is the provision of a reproducible, non-invasive study that is highly sensitive and specific and well tolerated by the patient. The optimal imaging strategy for staging patients with colorectal liver metastases for resection remains to be defined and depends to some degree on local resources and expertise and, crucially, on the availability of the imaging modalities [1].

2.2
Ultrasonography

2.2.1
Technique

Conventional transabdominal ultrasonography (US) is still used to detect the presence of liver metastases. Real-time trans-abdominal US offers a rapid and non-invasive technique for screening patients with suspected colorectal liver metastases. Conventional US is carried out using a curved 3.5-MHz transducer and conventional B-mode. The acoustic power usually is preset at a mechanical index (MI) of 0.08–0.18 (mean 0.10). The examination is performed in longitudinal and transversal planes of the liver, with the patient placed in the supine and oblique left position, respectively. Good scanning is obtained when the posterior and lateral surfaces of the liver are clearly visualized by a subcostal medioclavicular approach.

Contrast-enhanced US (CEUS), in which the patient is administered intravenous contrast media, seems to improve the sensitivity of detecting liver metastases. At present, CEUS is carried out following intravenous infusion of new-generation microbubble contrast agents (perfluorocarbon or sodium chloride gas stabilized by a protein, lipid, or polymer shell), which are detected using optimized imaging methods, i.e., a conventional US imager sends pulses into tissue at one frequency but selectively detects echoes at double that frequency (harmonic imaging). Microbubble contrast agents, which are purely intravascular, are well tolerated and allow for the sensitive real-time evaluation of blood flow in hepatic lesions. Patients receive a bolus infusion of a contrast agent in a peripheral vein immediately followed by a 5-ml saline flush to clear the infusion line and to prevent a decrease in the flow of contrast agent in the veins of the arm. CEUS is performed using contrast-specific imaging software at low acoustic power output (MI < 0.1). The liver is assessed in the arterial (15–35 s), portal-venous (40–120 s), and late (> 120 s) phases following the injection of contrast medium. Exploration of the liver is possible until a marked overall decrease in contrast signal intensity occurs or when the complete disappearance of contrast has been reached; the latter occurs, on average, 3–6 min after contrast injection [6].

2.2.2
Imaging Findings

Most colorectal liver metastases are round, oval, or lobulated hypoechoic areas with surrounding liver parenchyma (Fig. 2.1). The presence of a hypoechoic ring or calcifications is typical but not specific of liver metastasis. However, some metastases are difficult to detect: isoechoic metastases have the same or similar acoustic behavior as the surrounding normal liver tissue, while hyperechoic metastases mimic hemangiomas. It is well known that US sensitivity is reduced in patients with obesity, a high-lying diaphragm, interposition of the intestine, or who are uncooperative. However, US is helpful in characterizing indeterminate lesions discovered using other imaging modalities and provides a fast and effective guidance technique for biopsy [1]. After contrast injection, colorectal liver metastases present contrast washout in the portal-venous phase, thus becoming markedly hypoechoic or even anechoic in the late phase, regardless of the arterial phase pattern (Fig. 2.2) [6]. During the portal-venous phase, liver metastases typically enhance less than the liver, whereas benign lesions are more enhanced.

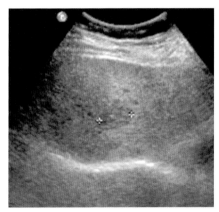

Fig. 2.1 A liver metastasis hypoechoic with surrounding liver parenchyma

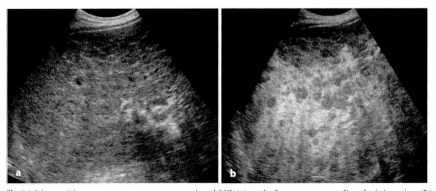

Fig. 2.2 Liver with metastases seen at conventional US (**a**) and after contrast media administration (**b**)

2.3
Computed Tomography

2.3.1
Technique

Computed tomography (CT) remains the mainstay of liver imaging and covers most of the clinical indications [7, 8], assessing both intra- and extra-hepatic disease extent. With the advent of multi-row detector (two and four) scanners in 1998, coverage of the liver within a single breath-hold of 10–14 s became feasible and decreased the likelihood of motion artifacts due to breathing during scanning. Multidetector-row CT (MDCT) is the most commonly used imaging modality for the detection and characterization of hepatic metastases [9]. Currently, MDCT scanners with 40–64 or more rows and a submillimetric detector configuration are available. Rotation time has decreased to 0.33 s with scanners of the latest generation, allowing the liver to be scanned with submillimeter collimation within a single breath-hold of no more than 2–3 s. Several studies have assessed the value of using thin slices to improve the detection of small metastases. In the study of Weg et al. [10], 2.5-mm-thick slices were significantly superior to 5-, 7.5-, and 10-mm-thick slices. In the study of Kopka et al. [11], a slice thickness of 3.75 mm proved superior to 5-mm-thick slices in terms of lesion characterization, and to those with a thickness of 7.5 mm in terms of detection and characterization. A decrease of the slice thickness to 1 mm does not result in further improvement in lesion detection but there is a considerable increase in image noise, with subsequent degradation of image quality [12]. Therefore, a slice thickness of 2–4 mm is recommended for axial viewing. Not surprisingly, differences between imaging protocols are most prominent when small liver lesions (< 10 mm) are evaluated [11]. Visualization of liver lesions is improved by contrast injection; in fact, contrast agent enables a better detection of colorectal liver metastases based on differences in uptake by the different tissues. Moreover, helical scanning combined with faster, powered iodine contrast injection (3–5 ml/s) enables the entire liver to be evaluated in specific vascular phases [1].

The liver should be examined in a standardized manner by an unenhanced scan performed primarily to characterize small lesions as being solid or cystic and to detect calcified lesions. Then, an intravenous contrast-enhanced study is carried out using a non-ionic iodine contrast agent (with a dose of 100–150 ml, according to iodine concentration and patient weight) administered in a peripheral vein with a flow-rate of 3–5 ml/s. The following phases are usually performed after contrast injection: late arterial phase (30–35 s), portal-venous phase (after 55–70 s), and delayed phase (after 180 s). The late arterial phase is useful to detect hypervascular lesions, while the portal-venous phase allows the detection of hypovascular lesions [1]. Dual-phase evaluation, with late arterial and portal-venous phases, has improved the detection and characterization of hypervascular lesions [13]. It has also increased the detection of hypovascular colorectal metastases, although studies have shown that it does not alter surgical management [14, 15]. Delayed images are essential to differentiate between hemangioma and metastases; the latter may show peripheral enhancement but sometimes may exhibit a central fill-in phenomenon, a feature mostly seen in hemangioma.

An early arterial phase (within 20 s after intravenous bolus injection) may be useful in demonstrating hepatic arterial anatomy for surgical planning but is of little value in the detection and characterization of liver metastases. In addition to the 2- to 4-mm-thick slices obtained for viewing, submillimeter slices are acquired for 3D image reconstructions. MDCT scanners have the capability to obtain high-resolution studies with submillimeter slice thickness, resulting in isotropic pixel sizes, that enable images to be reformatted in various planes with the same resolution as the axial images (Fig. 2.3). This may improve the detection of small lesions. High-resolution scans with maximum intensity technique and volumetric three-dimensional rendering enable the accurate segmental localization and delineation of tumor [16]. Vascular reconstruction demonstrates the hepatic arterial and portal-venous anatomy, obviating the need for conventional angiography in the surgical planning of tumor resection (Fig. 2.4) [17]. Volumetric measurement of tumor size and normal liver is

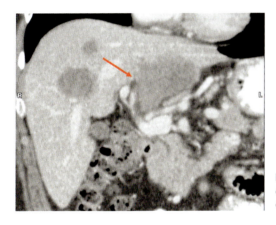

Fig. 2.3 A reformatted coronal CT image demonstrating portal invasion by a liver metastasis (*red arrow*)

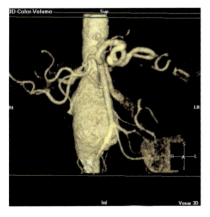

Fig. 2.4 Vascular reconstruction demonstrates that the right hepatic artery arises from the superior mesenteric artery

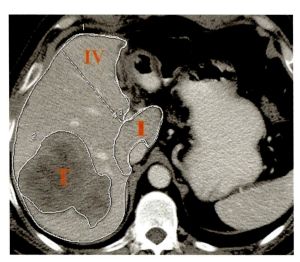

Fig. 2.5 Area measurement of tumor size and normal liver on a CT image is useful in performing CT volumetry. *T*, tumor; *I*, segment I; *IV*, segment IV

also more accurate [18]. CT volumetry is routinely performed when major liver resection is planned, in order to schedule preoperative portal-vein embolization when necessary (see Chapter 8, "Therapeutic Strategies in Unresectable Colorectal Liver Metastases"). MDCT technology provides high-speed and thin-section imaging of the entire volume during a single breath-hold and has proved to be an accurate method for the assessment of liver volumes (Fig. 2.5) [19].

2.3.2
Imaging Findings

The majority of colorectal liver metastases are solid hypovascular lesions. In the portal-venous phase, metastases become more conspicuous as lesions that are hypodense compared to normal liver. Late arterial phase imaging has been reported to improve lesion characterization of colorectal liver metastases, particularly lesions < 1 cm in diameter. Liver metastases may have a peripheral, circumferential rim enhancement due to increased perilesional blood vessels (Fig. 2.6) [20]. However, some colorectal liver metastases are hypervascular and appear hyperdense with respect to the surrounding liver in the late arterial phase. In fact, this phase is important, as mentioned above, in the diagnosis of hypervascular metastases and in the differentiation between these lesions and hemangiomas, especially in case of early and completely enhancing hemangiomas. Liver metastases are calcified in 11% of patients at initial presentation [21]. These lesions are much better seen on unenhanced scans than on portal-venous phase scans.

2 Diagnosis and Staging

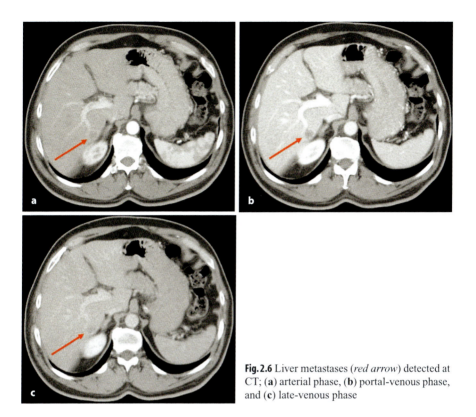

Fig. 2.6 Liver metastases (*red arrow*) detected at CT; (**a**) arterial phase, (**b**) portal-venous phase, and (**c**) late-venous phase

2.4 Magnetic Resonance Imaging

2.4.1 Technique

Magnetic resonance imaging (MRI) has become established as an important imaging modality in the detection and characterization of colorectal liver metastases. MRI is performed on a 1.5- to 3-Tesla system using a phased-array body coil and high-performance gradient. Routine breath-hold unenhanced T1-weighted sequences and breath-hold T2-weighted axial imaging sequences of the liver, with or without fat suppression, are performed. Magnetic resonance contrast agents have been developed to improve the detection and characterization of liver lesions. They are classified as extracellular, reticuloendothelial, hepatobiliary, blood pool, and combined agents.

The most commonly used agents for liver imaging are low-molecular-weight gadolinium (Gd) chelates belonging to the class of extracellular agents. They make it possible to carry out multiphase hepatic MRI studies of the arterial and venous phases, thus rendering a detailed map of the intrahepatic vascular tree and providing some degree of characterization of the different lesions according to their different blood supply and wash-out behaviors. However, the differences in signal intensity between a focal lesion and the surrounding normal parenchyma obtained using these extracellular agents are not always optimal. To overcome the limitations of low-molecular-weight Gd chelates, a new class of contrast agents has been developed specifically for liver imaging. The two main groups of contrast agents in this liver-specific class are superparamagnetic iron oxides (SPIO), taken up via the reticuloendothelial system mainly into the liver and spleen, and hepatobiliary contrast agents, taken up mainly by the hepatocytes and largely excreted via the bile ducts (Fig. 2.7). Three hepatobiliary contrast agents have been approved for clinical use and are commercially available: mangafodipir trisodium (Teslacan; GE Healthcare Milwaukee, WI, USA), gadobenate dimeglumine (MultiHance; Bracco Imaging S.p.a., Milan Italy), and gadoxate (Primovist; Bayer Schering Pharma AG, Berlin, Germany). Although these agents differ in their characterization and detection of various liver lesions [3], all of them produce a strong increase in the signal intensity of the liver,

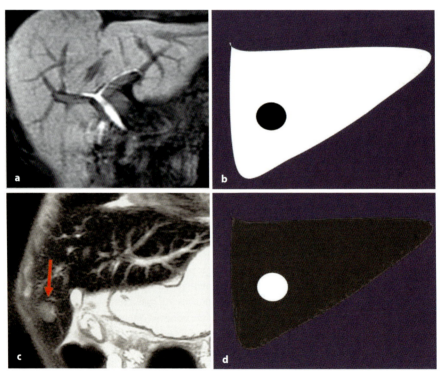

Fig. 2.7 a Hepatobiliary contrast agents excreted by the biliary system. **b** With hepatobiliary contrast agents metastatic lesions appear hypointense on T1-weighted imaging: scheme. **c** Superparamagnetic iron oxides taken up via the reticuloendothelial system. **d** With superparamagnetic iron oxides liver metastatic lesions appear hyperintense on T2-weighted imaging: scheme

bile ducts, and some hepatocyte-containing lesions on T1-weighted imaging [22]. Diffusion-weighted MRI (DWI) is sensitive to the molecular diffusion of water in biological tissues, and recent advancements have enabled high-quality DWI images of the liver to be obtained [23]. DWI is carried out using a breath-hold single-shot echo-planar (EPI) technique with parallel imaging and could be useful in detecting liver metastases. Apart from the visual assessment of liver metastases that is possible with EPI-DWI, the apparent diffusion coefficient can be quantitatively measured. The acquisition of unenhanced sequences and DWI are followed by the administration of hepatobiliary contrast agent (e.g., gadoxate), with multiphase hepatic MRI studies in the arterial, portal-venous, and hepatobiliary phases starting after 20 min.

2.4.2
Imaging Findings

Generally, colorectal liver metastases are hypointense on unenhanced T1-weighted images and slightly hyperintense and inhomogeneous on T2-weighted scans; after the administration of extracellular contrast agents, their appearance is similar to that on CT (Fig. 2.8). Most liver metastases are well detected during the portal-venous phase as lesions hypointense to the surrounding liver, with a rim of peripheral enhancement that is more evident on arterial phase. Regularly, metastases show a lack of Kupffer cells and a constant signal on T2-weighted accumulation phase images with SPIO particles. The superparamagnetic action causes increased spin dephasing and results in a significant reduction in normal liver signal intensities, most prominent on T2-weighted images, while metastases do not take up SPIO particles and thus appear hyperintense.

Lesion-to-liver contrast is significantly improved by the administration of hepatobiliary contrast agents, resulting in higher detection rates than is the case with conventional imaging techniques (Fig. 2.9). These agents, taken up by hepatocytes and largely excreted via the bile ducts, are not accumulated by liver lesions, which therefore appear strongly hypointense compared to the surrounding hyperintense liver. On

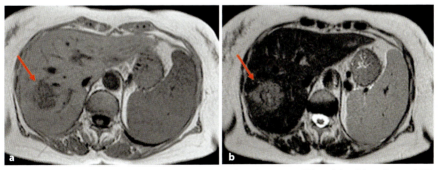

Fig. 2.8 Colorectal liver metastasis (*red arrow*) is (**a**) hypointense on T1-weighted imaging and (**b**) hyperintense on T2-weighted imaging

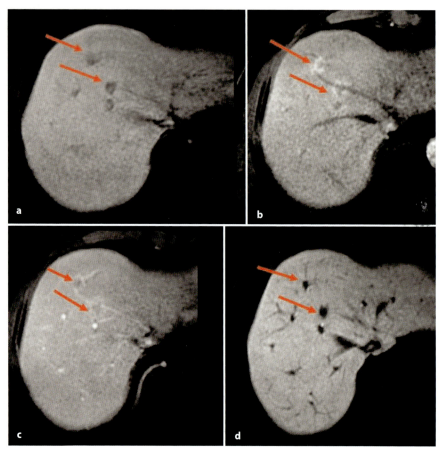

Fig. 2.9 Liver metastases (*red arrows*) detected after injection of gadoxate (Primovist), an extracellular and hepatobiliary contrast agent: (**a**) arterial phase, (**b**) portal-venous phase, (**c**) late venous phase, and (**d**) hepatobiliary phase. Lesion-to-liver contrast is improved in the last phase

DWI, colorectal hepatic metastases show high signal and restricted diffusion compared with normal liver parenchyma (Fig. 2.10).

2.5
Performance and Comparison of Imaging Modalities

Conventional US sensitivity is lower (53–77%) [6] than that of CT (85%) or intraoperative US (95%) [24]. In a recent meta-analysis [4] of five trials based on a per-patient analysis, US pooled sensitivity and specificity were 63% and 97%, ranging from 25% to 87% and from 95% to 100% (Table 2.1). US sensitivity depends on the

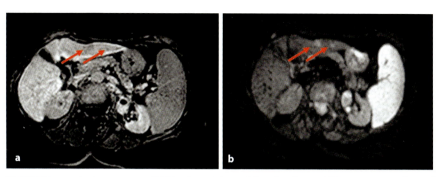

Fig. 2.10 Liver metastases seen on DWI as hyperintense (**a**) and on hepatobiliary contrast-enhanced MRI as hypointense (**b**); in combination, these sequences are helpful in identifying lesions

Table 2.1 Sensitivity and specificity of imaging modalities in the meta-analysis by Floriani et al. [4] on a per-patient and per-lesion basis

	Per patient		Per lesion	
	Sensitivity	Specificity	Sensitivity	Specificity
US	63% (25–87%)	97.6% (95–100%)	86.3%	
CT	74.8% (48.4–100%)	95.6% (80–100%)	82.6% (60–100%)	82.6% (60–100%)
MR	81.1% (64.3–100%)	97.2% (90.6–98.4%)	86.3% (64.3–100%)	87.2% (81.3–90.5%)
FDG-PET	93.8% (77.8–100%)	98.7% (96–100%)	86% (53.5–95.5%)	97.2% (80–98.7%)

echogenicity and size of the metastasis, decreasing to 20% for metastases < 10 mm. Recent studies have shown that CEUS improves sensitivity in detecting liver metastases from 63 to 91% and specificity from 60 to 88% [25]. These promising results are similar to the best-reported results of CT. However, most studies have included patients with established metastases [26] or selected patients with a high risk of metastases, probably leading to a greater accuracy than in unselected patients. Furthermore, some of the previous studies included a small number of patients or did not have a clear gold standard [25, 26]. At present, CEUS does not replace CT and MRI in the preoperative screening of colorectal liver metastases, due to limitations such as scanning condition, observer dependence, and problems comparing long video sequences at follow-up [6, 24, 27].

The use of MDCT was shown to improve resolution and increase the sensitivity of detecting liver metastases up to 70–90%. Nowadays, MDCT is the mainstay of staging and follow-up of these patients, as it provides good coverage of the liver and the entire abdomen and chest in one session. In a recent meta-analysis [4], CT was tested in 12 trials based on a per-patient analysis. The pooled sensitivity and specificity were 74.8% and 95.6%, ranging from 48.4% to 100% and from 80.0% to 100%, respectively. In the 17 studies [4] considering lesions as units of observation, sensitivity and specificity were 82.6% and 58.6%, ranging from 60.0% to 100% and 35.1% to 72.0%, respectively. The limitations of CT include its low sensitivity in detecting extrahepatic disease and subcentimeter hepatic lesions [28], missing up to 25% of liver metastases.

In a European phase 3 trial, mangafodipir-enhanced MRI identified a greater number of lesions than unenhanced MRI in 22–36% of patients; in the same study, in a comparison with contrast enhanced CT, mangafodipir-enhanced MRI identified a greater number of lesions in 31.1% of the cases and fewer lesions in 13.4% [14]. In a different phase 3 trial from the United States, mangafodipir-enhanced MRI was comparable or superior to CT [29]. One of the limits of both studies is that not all patients underwent spiral CT. There is evidence that mangafodipir-enhanced MRI is likely to influence the operative decision in candidates for surgical resection of liver metastases, by detecting small lesions not shown at CT scan. In 2004, Bartolozzi et al. [30] presented the results of a prospective, multi-institutional trial whose primary end-point was to compare the sensitivity of unenhanced and mangafodipir enhanced MRI with that of spiral CT in the detection of liver metastases from colorectal cancer. The authors used as the standard of reference intraoperative US (IOUS), which detected a total of 128 metastatic lesions, ranging from 0.2 to 12.0 cm in diameter. Forty-seven of the 128 lesions were ≤ 1 cm in diameter; 31 ranged from 1.1 to 2 cm, and 45 were > 2 cm. Histological confirmation of the metastases was obtained in the 89 of 128 lesions that were surgically removed; the remaining 39 lesions were subjected to intra-operative radiofrequency thermal ablation. Results from the per-lesion analysis showed an overall detection rate of 71% (91 of 128 lesions) for spiral CT, 72% (92 of 128) for unenhanced MRI, and 90% (115 of 128) for mangafodipir-enhanced MRI. The latter was significantly more sensitive than either unenhanced MRI ($p < 0.0001$) or spiral CT ($p = 0.0007$). The difference in sensitivity of mangafodipir-enhanced MRI vs. spiral CT and unenhanced MRI was even more significant for lesions ≤ 1 cm (Fig. 2.11). Finally, all lesions undetected by mangafodipir-enhanced MRI and discovered at the time of surgery by IOUS did not exceed 1 cm in diameter.

Kim et al. [31] evaluated 69 patients with colorectal cancer, finding a total of 181 liver lesions, benign and malignant, ranging from 0.2 to 12.5 cm in largest diameter. The detection rates of mangafodipir-enhanced MRI and helical CT did not significantly differ, whether considering all the hepatic lesions or only the metastases. However, if only small (≤ 2 cm) hepatic metastases were considered, the detection rate of mangafodipir-enhanced MRI was significantly higher than that of helical CT, both overall ($p = 0.022$) and compared to histopathologic confirmation ($p = 0.043$).

In our experience, mangafodipir is very accurate in detecting liver metastases in patients with colorectal cancer [32]. We reviewed the findings of spiral CT and mangafodipir-enhanced MRI in 125 consecutive patients undergoing surgery for colorectal cancer with or without liver metastases, in whom 192 lesions in total were detected. At least one liver metastasis was detected in 62 of the 125 patients; in the remaining 63 patients no lesions were detected at IOUS. Per-patient diagnostic accuracy and sensitivity in the detection of liver metastases from colorectal cancer were significantly higher for mangafodipir-enhanced MRI than for spiral CT, the difference

2 Diagnosis and Staging

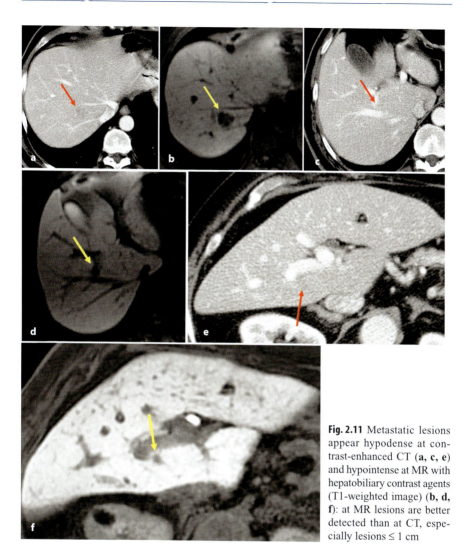

Fig. 2.11 Metastatic lesions appear hypodense at contrast-enhanced CT (**a, c, e**) and hypointense at MR with hepatobiliary contrast agents (T1-weighted image) (**b, d, f**): at MR lesions are better detected than at CT, especially lesions ≤ 1 cm

being most evident for lesions with a largest diameter ≤ 1 cm. In this group, spiral CT, unenhanced MRI, and enhanced MRI detected respectively 31 (48%), 35 (54%), and 44 (68%) of the 65 metastases.

2.6
Positron Emission Tomography

Positron emission tomography (PET) using [^{18}F]fluoro-2-deoxy-D-glucose (FDG) has recently emerged as a promising imaging modality in the staging of patients with recurrent or metastatic colorectal cancer [28]. The biological basis of FDG-PET is that tumors have higher glycolytic activity than non-cancerous tissues. Administration of the glucose analog FDG to a patient with cancer is followed by its transport into tumor cells via hexose (GLUT) transporters and its subsequent phosphorylation by the glycolytic enzyme hexokinase. Since FDG-6-phosphate cannot proceed down the glycolytic pathway, it selectively accumulates in the tumor, which can then be imaged based on the 511-keV photons released from bound fluorine-18. Although the tracer is not tumor-cell-specific (inflammatory tissues also take up FDG), FDG-PET is widely used in the diagnostic work-up of many malignant diseases [33], including colorectal cancer, because it provides functional characterization of lesions identified using a first-line imaging modality, such as CT, and more accurate definition of tumor extent by improving lesion detection, particularly for extrahepatic disease [34]. In addition to the potential for improved lesion detection, the intensity of FDG uptake, quantified by calculating the maximum standardized uptake value (SUV), may correlate with tumor behavior and patient outcome. In other malignancies, such as lung cancer and esophageal cancer, the intensity of FDG uptake is an independent predictor of clinical outcome and a useful parameter to assess patient response to preoperative treatments. A recent meta-analysis of publications determined an average sensitivity and specificity of FDG-PET of 88% and 96%, respectively, for detecting hepatic colorectal metastases. Corresponding figures for detecting extrahepatic disease are 90% and 95%, respectively. These results are impressive and have the potential to change the overall management plan in 20–25% of patients [35]. This improved patient selection may translate into longer postoperative survival. In a prospective study, Fernandez et al. [36] demonstrated a clear survival benefit when patients were stringently selected for liver surgery after screening with FDG-PET/CT for distant colorectal metastases. Their study reported a high 5-year post-resection survival rate (58%).

Conventional PET scanning, however, is associated with several shortcomings. Firstly, it is relatively insensitive in the detection of small and mucinous lesions. Reports indicate that 67–92% of hepatic metastases < 1 cm are not detected [37, 38]. This poor sensitivity in the liver results from both the relatively high FDG uptake of normal hepatocytes and the acquisition parameters used in standard scans that seek to perform a whole-body survey within a reasonable length of time. Secondly, at least two studies [37, 39] demonstrated a reduced sensitivity of mangafodipir-enhanced liver MRI and MDCT in detecting hepatic metastases subjected to chemotherapy (Tables 2.2 and 2.3). Akhurst et al. [38] showed that the number of undetected hepatic lesions was significantly higher in patients treated with preoperative chemotherapy (37%) than in those who did not receive preoperative treatment (23%). Notably, in patients undergoing upfront hepatic resection, no cancerous lesions > 1.2 cm were missed by PET. Conversely, when FDG-PET was used to evaluate patients undergoing concurrent chemotherapy, a lesion as large as 3.2 cm was missed. Similarly, Adie et al. [40] found that preoperative chemotherapy interferes with the mechanism of FDG-PET uptake, resulting in a lower sensitivity in chemotreated patients. Therefore, FDG uptake seems to be unreliable in patients with recent chemotherapy. Thirdly, the major drawback of PET images relates to the poor spatial resolution,

Table 2.2 Sensitivity and diagnostic accuracy of MnDPDP MRI and FDG PET in the detection of colorectal cancer liver metastases, as reported by Sahani et al. [17] on a per-patient basis and per-lesion basis[a]

	Per patient		Per lesion	
	Sensitivity	Diagnostic accuracy	Sensitivity	Diagnostic accuracy
MnDPDP MRI	96.6%	97.7%	81.4%	75.5%
FDG-PET	93.3%	85.3% (80–98.7%)	67%	64.1% (80–98.7%)

[a]MRI detected more hepatic metastases than FDG-PET ($p = 0.016$); all of the 33 lesions measuring < 1 cm and confirmed by the reference standard were identified by MRI, whereas only 12 were detected by FDG-PET ($p = 0.0001$)

Table 2.3 Sensitivity of FDG-PET and CT in patients treated with or without preoperative chemotherapy (from [37])

	Group 1	Group 2
PET sensitivity	93.3%	49%
CT sensitivity	87.5%	65.3%

Group 1, immediate hepatic resection; group 2, hepatic resection following neoadjuvant chemotherapy

making the exact localization of FDG uptake difficult. As a result, the diagnosis ultimately relies on a correlation between findings obtained on CT or MRI and the PET scan. To overcome this limitation, a new technique combining the same imaging session data of a full-ring PET-scanner with helical MDCT has been developed. With this novel technology, PET/CT, PET-positive lesions are projected directly onto the CT scan to obtain simultaneous functional and anatomic information, with a significant improvement in the localization and characterization of lesions, thus enabling an accurate definition of the extension of disease at the time of diagnosis [41]. Data indicate that the combination of CT and FDG-PET increases the sensitivity of lesion detection over PET alone from 75% to 89% [35]. A recent study on 467 patients compared the sensitivity, specificity, and diagnostic accuracy of single PET scan, single CT scan, and PET/CT scan [42]. The results were as follows: PET scan had 94.05% sensitivity, 91.6% specificity, and 93.36% accuracy; CT scan had 91.07% sensitivity, 95.42% specificity, and 92.29% accuracy; and PET/CT had 97.92% sensitivity, 97.71% specificity, and 97.86% accuracy.

In addition, PET/CT has proven particularly effective when, in the presence of a progressive increase in tumor markers, clinical or imaging techniques nonetheless fail to demonstrate disease recurrence. The PET/CT results lead to an earlier diagnosis, with a positive impact on patient survival. The change in FDG uptake in fact correlates with serum carcinoembryonic antigen (CEA) levels. increased CEA levels are a common finding in these patients. Moreover, use of PET/CT leads to an overall reduction in costs compared to the separate use of the two imaging modalities. A cost-benefit analysis performed in the United States and Europe showed that PET/CT enables improved patient selection for surgery and, as a result, is cost effective. Lastly, by optimizing study protocols, the combined PET/CT examination reduces the overall dose of radiation delivered to the patient and the overall examination time, thus minimizing patient discomfort. Whether to routinely use FDG-PET or PET/CT in the preoperative evaluation of patients with suspected or proven hepatic colorectal metastases is still controversial. Where economic factors play a limiting role, PET/CT can be selectively directed toward patients with higher risk of tumor recurrence, such as patients with multiple or synchronous metastases, as the probability of obtaining a result that will affect management increases in this population.

2.7
Diagnosis and Staging of Liver Metastases from Colorectal Cancer

Nowadays, MDCT is the mainstay of staging and follow-up of patients with colorectal cancer because in one session it provides good coverage of the liver, the complete abdomen, and the chest.

Due to restricted availability and high cost, FDG-PET and PET/CT should be used in selected patients in whom the diagnosis is not clear following conventional diagnostic modalities, or in selected high-risk patients.

In patients with potentially resectable liver metastases, preoperative liver evaluation by MRI with a hepatospecific contrast agent is indicated.

Staging with IOUS is more accurate than preoperative evaluation with CT and MRI. The findings obtained by IOUS changed the surgical strategy in 22.8% of patients who underwent preoperative tumor staging with MDCT and MRI without the use of extracellular agents [43]. A recent study by Tamandl et al. [44] evaluated the role of contrast-enhanced MDCT and MRI with specific agents in the preoperative assessment of patients with liver metastases, giving a different perspective on the role of imaging in surgical planning. The authors reviewed data from 194 consecutive liver resections in patients with liver metastases from colorectal cancer, with a total of 408 lesions; MDCT and MRI with a hepatospecific agent (either mangafodipir or gadoxate) were performed in all patients prior to surgery. Images were routinely evaluated and reviewed by attending radiologists with extensive expertise in hepatobiliary diagnostics, and the results were regularly discussed at weekly multidisciplinary meetings with liver surgeons, medical oncologists, radiologists, and radiation oncologists. Additional lesions were detected intraoperatively in only 16 of the 194 patients (8.2%); in 11 cases (5.7%), the lesions were < 1 cm and subcapsular. The authors concluded that preoperative imaging with contrast-enhanced total-body MDCT and MRI with a liver-specific contrast agent is efficient and very seldom leads to a change in the surgical strategy, and that patients with additional resectable liver metastases have a higher risk of recurrence and should be monitored carefully.

2.8
Liver Metastases Detection After Chemotherapy

The detection of liver metastases at CT is more difficult following chemotherapy [37]. Although this may be due to the fact that the lesions have decreased in size and are less conspicuous, there is also the possibility that they become difficult to detect because of drug-induced steatosis, which modifies the density of the normal liver parenchyma (Fig. 2.12).

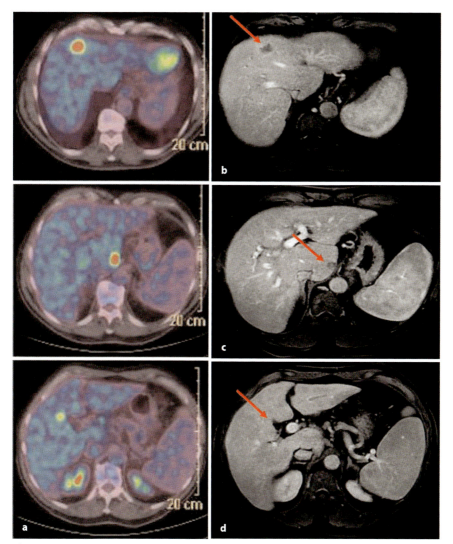

Fig. 2.12 Liver metastases detected at PET/CT (**a**) and at contrast-enhanced MRI (*arrows*, **b, c, d**) after the administration of Gd chelates

One of the potential applications of contrast-enhanced MRI is to assess the extent of metastatic liver disease in patients who have received neoadjuvant chemotherapy. We recently evaluated the diagnostic accuracy of spiral CT and mangafodipir-enhanced MRI in detecting liver metastases from colorectal cancer in a series of patients undergoing surgery following neoadjuvant chemotherapy [45]. The study group comprised 36 patients (14 females and 22 males, median age 61 years) with a total of 132 lesions. The standard of reference was the histology of the surgically excised lesions, or IOUS in cases in which pathological assessment was not possible. We used a 16-slice CT scanner and a 1.5-Tesla MRI unit. The per-lesion sensitivity, specificity, and accuracy were, respectively, 64.5% (69/107), 36% (9/25), and 59.1% (78/132) for CT, and 83.2% (89/107), 40% (10/25), and 75% (99/132) for mangafodipir-enhanced MRI. Sensitivity and accuracy were significantly higher for MRI with tissue-specific agent than with CT ($p = 0.0023$ and $p < 10^{-3}$, respectively).

The potential role of DWI in the in the assessment of disease response to novel therapeutics, including anti-vascular and anti-angiogenic therapy, must still be evaluated [46].

References

1. Ong KO, Leen E (2007) Radiological staging of colorectal liver metastases. Surg Oncol 16:7-14
2. Simmonds PC, Primrose JN, Colquitt JL et al (2006) Surgical resection of hepatic metastases from colorectal cancer: a systematic review of published studies. Br J Cancer 94: 982-999
3. Regge D, Cirillo S, Macera A et al (2009) Mangafodipir trisodium: review of its use as an injectable contrast medium for magnetic resonance imaging. Reports in Medical Imaging 2:55-68
4. Floriani I, Torri V, Rulli E et al (2010) Performance of imaging modalities in diagnosis of liver metastases from colorectal cancer: a Systematic review and meta-analysis. J Magn Reson Imaging 31:19-31
5. Simmonds PC (2000) Palliative chemotherapy for advanced colorectal cancer: systematic review and meta-analysis. Colorectal Cancer Collaborative Group. British Medical Journal 321:531-535
6. Larsen LPS, Rosenkilde M, Christensen H et al (2007) The value of contrast enhanced ultrasonography in detection of liver metastases from colorectal cancer: a prospective double-blinded study. Eur J Radiol 62:302-307
7. Scott DJ, Guthrie JA, Arnold P et al (2001) Dual phase helical CT versus portal venous phase CT for the detection of colorectal liver metastases: correlation with intra-operative sonography, surgical and pathological findings. Clinical Radiol 56:235–242
8. Bluemke DA, Paulson EK, Choti MA et al (2000) Detection of hepatic lesions in candidates for surgery: comparison of ferumoxides-enhanced MR imaging and dualphase helical CT. Am J Roentgenol 175:1653–1658
9. Schima W, Kulinna C, Langenberger H et al (2005) Liver metastases of colorectal cancer: US, CT or MR? Cancer Imaging. Spec No A:S149-56
10. Weg N, Scheer MR, Gabor MP (1998) Liver lesions: improved detection with dual-detector-array CT and routine 2.5-mm thin collimation. Radiology 209:417–26
11. Kopka L, Grabbe E (1999) Biphasische Leberdiagnostik mit der Mehrzeilendetektor-Spiral-CT. Radiologe 39:971–978

12. Kulinna C, Helmberger T, Kessler M et al (2001) Verbesserung der Diagnostik von Lebermetastasen mit der Multi-Detektor-CT. Radiologe 41:16–23
13. Van Hoe L, Baert AL, Gryspeerdt S (1997) Dual-phase helical CT of the liver: value of an early-phase acquisition in the differential diagnosis of noncystic focal lesions. Am J Roentgenol 168:1185–1192
14. Padovani B, Lecesne R, Raffaelli C et al (1996) Tolerability and utility of mangafodipir trisodium injection (MnDPDP) at the dose of 5 μmol/kg body weight in detecting focal liver tumors: results of a phase III trial using an infusion technique. Eur J Radiol 23:205–211
15. Gearhart SL, Frassica D, Rosen R et al (2006) Improved staging with pretreatment positron emission tomography/computed tomography in low rectal cancer. Ann Surg Oncol 13:397–404
16. Kamel IR, Georgiades C, Fishman EK (2003) Incremental value of advanced image processing of multislice computed tomography data in the evaluation of hypervascular liver lesions. J Comp Assisted Tomography 27:652–656
17. Sahani D, Mehta A, Blake M et al (2004) Preoperative hepatic vascular evaluation with CT and MR angiography: implications for surgery. Radiographics 24:1367–1380
18. Yim PJ, Vora AV, Raghavan D et al (2006) Volumetric analysis of liver metastases in computed tomography with the fuzzy C-means algorithm. J Comp Assisted Tomography 30:212–220
19. Zappa M, Dondero F, Sibert A et al (2009) Liver regeneration at day 7 after right hepatectomy: global and segmental volumetric analysis by using CT. Radiology 252:426-432
20. Freeny PC, Gardner JC, von Ingersleben G et al (1995) Hepatic helical CT: effect of reduction of iodine dose of intravenous contrast material on hepatic contrast enhancement. Radiology 197:89–93
21. Hale HL, Husband JE, Gossios K et al (1998) CT of calcified liver metastases in colorectal cancer. Clin Radiol 53:735–741
22. Gandhi SN, Brown MB, Wong JG et al (2006) MR contrast agents for liver imaging: what, when, how. Radiographics 6:1621–1636
23. Koh DM, Brown G, Riddell AM et al (2008) Detection of colorectal hepatic metastases using MnDPDP MR imaging and diffusion-weighted imaging (DWI) alone and in combination. Eur Radiol 18:903–910
24. Scott DJ, Guthrie JA, Arnold P et al (2001) Dual phase helical CT versus portal venous phase CT for the detection of colorectal liver metastases: correlation with intra-operative sonography, surgical and pathological findings. Clin Radiol 56:235–242
25. Albrecht T, Blomley MJ, Burns PN et al (2003) Improved detection of hepatic metastases with pulse-inversion US during the liver-specific phase of SHU 508A: multicenter study. Radiology 227:361–370
26. Quaia E, D'Onofrio M, Palumbo A et al (2006) Comparison of contrast-enhanced ultrasonography versus baseline ultrasound and contrast-enhanced computed tomography in metastatic disease of the liver: diagnostic performance and confidence. Eur Radiol 16:1599–1609
27. Larsen LPS, Rosenkilde M, Christensen H et al (2009) Can contrast-enhanced ultrasonography replace multidetector-computed tomography in the detection of liver metastases from colorectal cancer? Eur J Radiol 69:308-313
28. Sharma S, Camci C, Jabbour N (2008) Management of hepatic metastasis from colorectal cancers: an update. J Hepatobiliary Pancreat Surg 15:570-580
29. Federle MP, Chezmar JL, Rubin DL et al (2000) Safety and efficacy of mangafodipir trisodium (MnDPDP) injection for hepatic MRI in adults: results of the US multicenter phase III clinical trials. Efficacy of early imaging. J Magn Reson Imaging 12:689–701
30. Bartolozzi C, Donati F, Cioni D et al (2004) Detection of colorectal liver metastases: a prospective multi center trial comparing unenhanced MRI, MnDPDP-enhanced MRI, and spiral CT. Eur Radiol 14:14–20
31. Kim KW, Kim AY, Kim TK et al (2004) Small (<2 cm) hepatic lesion in colorectal cancer pa-

tients: detection and characterization on mangafodipir trisodium-enhanced MRI. Am J Roentgenol 14:14–20

32. Regge D, Campanella D, Anselmetti GC et al (2006) Diagnostic accuracy of portal phase CT and MRI with Mangafodipir trisodium in detecting liver metastases from colorectal carcinoma. Clin Rad 61:338–347

33. Lai CH, Yen TC, Chang TC (2007) Positron emission tomography imaging for gynecologic malignancy. Curr Opin Obstet Gynecol 19:37-41

34. Rohren EM, Turkington TG, Coleman RE (2004) Clinical applications of PET in oncology. Radiology 231:305–332

35. Wiering B, Krabbe PF, Jager GJ et al (2005) The impact of fluorine-18-deoxyglucose-positron emission tomography in the management of colorectal liver metastases. Cancer 104:2658-2670

36. Fernandez FG, Drebin JA, Linehan DC et al (2004) Five-year survival after resection of hepatic metastases from colorectal cancer in patients screened by positron emission tomography with F-18 fluorodeoxyglucose (FDG-PET). Ann Surg 240:438–447

37. Lubezky N, Metser U, Geva R et al (2007) The role and limitations of 18-fluoro-2-deoxy-D-glucose positron emission tomography (FDG-PET) scan and computerized tomography (CT) in restaging patients with hepatic colorectal metastases following neoadjuvant chemotherapy: comparison with operative and pathological findings. J Gastrointest Surg 11:472–478

38. Akhurst T, Kates TJ, Mazumdar M et al (2005) Recent chemotherapy reduces the sensitivity of [18F]fluorodeoxyglucose positron emission tomography in the detection of colorectal metastases. J Clin Oncol 23:8713-8716

39. Sahani DV, Kalva SP, Fischman AJ et al (2005) Detection of liver metastases from adenocarcinoma of the colon and pancreas. Comparison of MnDPDP liver MRI and whole body FDG PET. Am J Roengenol 185:239–246

40. Adie S, Yip C, Chu F, Morris DL (2009) Resection of liver metastases from colorectal cancer: does preoperative chemotherapy affect the accuracy of PET in preoperative planning? ANZ J Surg 79:358–361

41. Abdalla EK, Barnett CC, Doherty D et al (2002) Extended hepatectomy in patients with hepatobiliary malignancies with and without preoperative portal vein embolization. Arch Surg 137:675–680

42. Orlacchio A, Schillaci O, Fusco N et al (2009) Role of PET/CT in the detection of liver metastases from colorectal cancer. Radiol med 114:571-585

43. Zacherl J, Scheuba C, Imhof M et al (2002) Current value of intraoperative sonography during surgery for hepatic neoplasms. World J Surg 26:550-554

44. Tamandl D, Herberger B, Gruenberger B et al (2008) Adequate preoperative staging rarely leads to a change of intraoperative strategy in patients undergoing surgery for colorectal cancer liver metastases. Surgery 143:648–657

45. Gallo T, Cirillo S, Macera A et al (2009) To compare the diagnostic accuracy of portal-phase CT and MRI with mangafodipir trisodium in detection colorectal carcinoma following neoadjuvant therapy. [oral presentation] - ESGAR, June 23–26, Valencia

46. Koh DM, Scurr E, Collins DJ et al (2006) Colorectal hepatic metastases: quantitative measurements using single-shot echo planar diffusion-weighted MR imaging. Eur Radiol 16:1898-1905

Evolution of Resectability Criteria

3

Abstract Surgical resection is the gold standard in the treatment of colorectal liver metastases. Extension of the indications has, not surprisingly, determined an increase in the recurrence rates, underlining the need for appropriate selection of those patients who may benefit most from surgery. However, literature data suggest that the presence of any combination of pre-operative factors should not be used as an absolute contraindication to resection. Instead, colorectal liver metastases should be treated by resection whenever liver resection is technically feasible, with curative intent.

3.1
Introduction

The value of hepatic resection for colorectal liver metastases has never been demonstrated in prospective randomized trials. Nevertheless, it must be recognized that non-surgical treatment has never achieved long-term survival rates comparable with those reported by many non-randomized surgical series [1, 2]. In a famous paper published in 1990, Scheele analyzed the long-term outcome of three groups of patients with liver metastases: group 1 consisted of 902 patients with unequivocally unresectable disease, group 2 had 62 patients with resectable but not- resected disease (due to different therapeutic approaches at that time), and group 3 comprised 173 patients treated by resection. Since no patients from groups 1 and 2 were alive at 5 years vs. 25 (15%) in group 3, Scheele concluded that radical excision of colorectal liver metastases could offer effective "palliation" and, in a small number of patients, the chance of cure [3]. Today, two decades after this paper, surgical resection has become the gold standard "curative" treatment for patients with resectable colorectal liver metastases, with mortality < 1% and 5-year survival rates of up to 58% [4, 5].

A. Muratore (✉)
Division of Hepato-Bilio-Pancreatic and Digestive Surgery, Mauriziano "Umberto I" Hospital, Turin, Italy

Surgical Treatment of Colorectal Liver Metastases. Lorenzo Capussotti (Ed.)
© Springer-Verlag Italia 2011

3.2
Resectability Criteria

Preoperative selection of the best candidates for liver surgery depends on two factors: general medical fitness and disease extent. Anesthesiologists should identify and exclude from surgery patients at high operative risk (e.g., those with severe chronic obstructive pulmonary disease or congestive heart failure) while patients with manageable comorbidities may have their conditions proactively addressed in order to reduce the surgical risk.

Tumor resectability criteria have changed over time. In 1986, Ekberg stated that liver resection for colorectal liver metastases was indicated only if three prerequisites were satisfied: no more than three liver metastases, clear resection margin of ≥ 10 mm, and absence of extrahepatic disease [6]. Similar ground rules were reported a few years later by Steele, from Harvard Medical School [7]. However, as the safety of liver resections has improved, advanced surgical techniques (e.g., two-step hepatectomy) have been introduced, and new efficient chemotherapy regimens have become available, liver surgeons have assumed an increasingly aggressive attitude towards the management of hepatic colorectal metastases. Indeed, the overall rate of patients undergoing resection either for single or metachronous colorectal liver metastases decreased from 71% in two series of the 1980s to only 45% in a recent series [2, 8, 9]. Moreover, in a recent French study, only 24 (18%) of 131 patients who underwent liver resection for colorectal metastases also had resection of their extrahepatic disease [10]. The favorable long-term results of this aggressive surgical policy, combined with efficient peri-operative chemotherapy, challenges these ground rules; however, an extension of the indications has clearly increased the recurrence rates. In our series, recurrence after curative resection of colorectal liver metastases increased significantly with the extension of indications: 94% in patients with initially unresectable disease who were down-staged to surgery after neoadjuvant chemotherapy vs. 66% in patients with immediately resectable disease ($p = 0.001$) [5]. Thereafter, the issue of appropriate selection of stage IV patients who would most benefit from an aggressive approach has become increasingly important. Reporting the results of a survey conducted among members of the Association Francaise de Chirurgie, Nordlinger showed that age, stage of the primary tumor, size and number of the liver metastases, carcinoembryonic antigen (CEA) serum level, disease-free interval, and resection margin width were independent prognostic factors; these risk factors were used to establish a scoring system stratifying patients in three survival-risk groups [11]. Similarly, Fong analyzed a database of 1001 consecutive patients who underwent resection and identified five clinical criteria (lymph node status of the primary tumor, disease-free interval, number and size of liver metastases, CEA serum level) that were used to develop a clinical risk score [12]. However, these scores, if applied on a widespread basis, should be used cautiously, as they can result in the inappropriate denial of liver resection for those patients judged to be at high risk. It must be kept in mind that the 15–25% 5-year survival rate of high risk score patients, despite being lower than the 50–60% of low risk score patients, is certainly better than the 0% expected in similar patients without resection. Moreover, long-term survival is possible despite the presence of poor prognostic factors: in our series, one third of the patients who were alive 10 years after liver surgery had synchronous disease [13]. In the series reported from the Memorial Sloan-Kettering Cancer Center, more than one-third of the 96 patients with 5-year survival after liver resection for colorectal metastases had either multiple liver metastases or a short disease-free interval [14]. In Minagawa's study, most of the resected patients had synchronous, multiple liver metastases and Dukes C primary tumors: the 5-year survival rate was around 30%, with a median survival of 3 years [15]. The same presence of extrahepatic metastases (e.g., hepatic pedicle lymph node metastases or peritoneal carcinomatosis) is no longer an absolute contraindication to liver surgery as long as the liver disease is amenable to complete resection [16, 17]. Thereafter, any combination of preoperative prognostic factors should be used not to deny liver surgery but to enroll high-risk patients in trials of peri-operative chemotherapy. However, Adam et al. reported that tumor progression in patients on neoadjuvant chemotherapy for resectable colorectal liver metastases should be considered an absolute contraindication to liver resection since it is associated with a poor outcome (8% at 5 years) [10]. More recently, data analyzed from the LiverMetSurvey international registry confirmed that tumor progression during chemotherapy is a negative prognostic factor but not an absolute contraindication to liver resection: the 5-year survival rate after liver resection was 35% in the progression group vs. 50% in the non-progression group ($p = 0.002$) [18]. Similar findings were recently reported by Neumann et al. [19].

Currently, the indication for resection of liver metastases is determined by two factors. The first consists of the technical feasibility of the operation, which essentially depends on the location and the relationship of the liver metastases with vascular structures (e.g., hepatic veins), on the status of the underlying liver parenchyma (i.e., non-alcoholic fatty liver disease or sinusoidal dilatation by oxaliplatin-/irinotecan-based chemotherapy), and, if a major hepatic resection is planned, on the volume of the future liver remnant (FLR) (Fig. 3.1). A safe FLR obviously depends on the status of the underlying liver parenchyma; if the underlying liver is normal, a preoperative FLR > 25% seems to be safe, whereas if the liver is injured the preoperative FLR should be > 31–40% [20, 21]. The second factor is the possibility to obtain clear resection margins.

Over time, the conventional indications for surgical therapy of colorectal liver metastases have given way to more aggressive indications (Table 3.1). Currently, according to the conclusions of the Consensus Conference of the America Hepato-Pancreato-Biliary Association, colorectal liver metastases should be considered resectable whenever the disease can be completely resected, two adjacents liver segments can be spared, adequate vascular inflow and outflow and biliary drainage can be preserved, and the FLR is sufficient [22].

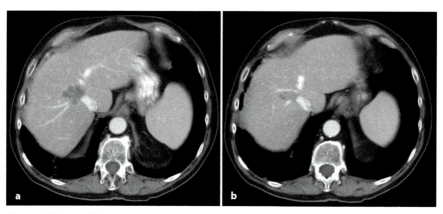

Fig. 3.1 a Colorectal liver metastases localized in Sg9 and (**b**) infiltrating the right hepatic vein and a branch to Sg8 of the middle hepatic vein. The planned operation is a right hepatectomy extended to Sg9. The remnant liver volume is 34%

Table 3.1 Conventional vs. modern indications for liver surgery of colorectal metastases

Conventional indications	Aggressive modern indications
≤ 3 liver metastases, unilobar	No limits for number or distribution (neoadjuvant chemotherapy, two-stage hepatectomy, radiofrequency ablation)
Size ≤ 5 cm	No size limits
No extrahepatic metastases	Resection of the extrahepatic disease (hepatic pedicle lymph-node metastases, local recurrence of the colorectal cancer, lung metastases)
Resection margin >1 cm	Negative resection margin
Adequate FRL	PVE or PVL in case of inadequate FLR
Metachronous metastases	Synchronous and metachronous metastases
No infiltration of IVC, hepatic veins, and hilar structures	No limits. Possible resection and/or reconstruction of vascular structures
Radical resection	

FLR, Future remnant liver; *IVC*, inferior vena cava; *PVE,* portal vein embolization; *PVL,* portal vein ligation

3.3
Resection Margin

There are no doubts that, in selecting patients for hepatic resection, the ability to achieve negative resection margins is mandatory since a positive margin after liver resection is correlated with significantly higher rates of surgical margin recurrence and worse long-term survival [9]. Nonetheless, it should be kept in mind that while achievement of a negative resection margin is mandatory when planning a hepatic resection, the problem is to define the minimum safe negative resection margin from an oncological point of view. For many years, a 1-cm negative margin was considered the gold standard and the inability to achieve it was often a contraindication to liver surgery [11, 23]. However, the increasing number of complex liver resections of multiple and bilateral metastases, especially if down-staged to surgery after neoadjuvant chemotherapy, has increased both the risk and the need to have negative but close resection margins. In the Adam's series, 81% of 335 patients with initially unresectable disease down-staged to surgery after neoadjuvant chemotherapy had a < 1-cm negative resection margin (0 mm in 67% of the patients) [24]. In 2005, a large multi-institutional series (M.D. Anderson Cancer Center, Houston, Texas; Ospedale Mauriziano "Umberto I", Torino, Italy; University Hospital, Geneva, Switzerland) of 557 patients showed that the width of a negative surgical resection margin affected neither recurrence nor survival rates [9]. A follow-up consensus conference of the American Hepato-Pancreato-Biliary Association confirmed the oncologic adequacy of a < 1 cm negative margin [25]. A more recent study from the Memorial Sloan-Kettering Cancer Center has re-ignited the debate by suggesting that a < 1 cm resection margin was an independent predictor of worse overall survival [26]. However, that study was problematic: first of all, the site of recurrence was not reported; second, the authors evaluated the prognostic significance of surgical margin width as a function not of recurrence-free survival but of overall survival time, which is heavily influenced by the type of treatment performed at the time of the metastasis recurrence. Two other studies reported that the surgical margin is an independent predictor of disease-free or hepatic-recurrence-free survival; however, the small number of patients in each subgroup of the Italian study and the different methods of liver parenchyma dissection of the German study, which might have caused misinterpretation of the resection margin, may have partially biased the results [27, 28]. A recent study from our group analyzed the impact of resection margin width on recurrence-free survival in 314 patients who underwent liver resection for colorectal metastases. Detailed pathologic analysis of the surgical margin was subsequently carried out together with complete follow-up imaging studies documenting disease status and site [29]. Node status of the primary tumor as well as the size and number of the metastases but not the width of the negative resection margin were independent prognostic factor of recurrence-free survival. Moreover, in support of this finding, most of the resection margin recurrences were associated with recurrences at other sites, usually intrahepatic.

In conclusion, a positive resection margin after potentially curative liver resection increases the risk of margin recurrence. Tumor biology and not the width of a negative resection margin influences recurrence-free survival.

References

1. Wagner JS, Adson MA, Van Heerden JA et al (1984) The natural history of hepatic metastases from colorectal cancer. A comparison with resective treatment. Ann Surg 199:502-507
2. Fortner JG, Silva JS, Golbey RB et al (1984) Multivariate analysis of a personal serie of 247 consecutive patients with liver metastases from colorectal cancer. Treatment by hepatic resection. Ann Surg 199:307-316
3. Scheele J, Stangl R, Altendorf-Hofmann A (1990) Hepatic metastases from colorectal carcinoma: impact of surgical resection on the natural history. Br J Surg 77:1241-1246
4. Abdalla EK, Vauthey JN, Ellis LM et al (2004) Recurrence and outcomes following hepatic resection, radiofrequency ablation, and combined resection/ablation for colorectal liver metastases. Ann Surg 239(6):818-825; discussion 825-827
5. Capussotti L, Muratore A, Mulas MM et al (2006) Neoadjuvant chemotherapy and resection for initially irresectable colorectal liver metastases. Br J Surg 93:1001-1006
6. Ekberg H, Tranberg JG, Andersson R et al (1986). Determinants of survival in liver resection for colorectal secondaries. Br J Surg 73:727-731
7. Steele G, Ravikumar TS (1989) Resection of hepatic metastases from colorectal cancer. Bioological perspectives. Ann Surg 212:127-138
8. Hughes KS, Rosenstein RB, Songhrabodi S et al (1988) Resection of the liver for colorectal carcinoma metastases. A multi-institutional study of long-term survivors. Dis Colon Rectum 31:1-4
9. Pawlik TM, Scoggins CR, Zorzi D et al (2005) Effect of surgical margin status on survival and site of recurrence after hepatic resection for colorectal metastases. Ann Surg 241:715-724
10. Adam R, Pascal G, Castaing D et al (2004). Tumor progression while on chemotherapy. A contraindication to liver resection for multiple colorectal metastases? Ann Surg 240:1052-1064
11. Nordlinger B, Guiguet M, Balladur P et al (1996) Surgical resection of colorectal carcinoma metastases to the liver. A prognostic scoring system to improve case selection, based on 1568 patients. Cancer 77:1254-1262
12. Fong Y, Fortner J, Sun RL et al (1999) Clinical score for predicting recurrence after hepatic resection for metastatic colorectal cancer. Analysis of 1001 consecutive cases. Ann Surg 230:309-321
13. Viganò L, Ferrero A, Lo Tesoriere R et al (2008) Liver surgery for colorectal liver metastases: results after 10 years of follow up. Long-term survivors, late recurrences, and prognostic role of morbidity. Ann Surg Oncol 15:2458-2464
14. D'Angelica M, Brennan MF, Fortner JG et al (1997) Ninety-six five-year survivors after liver resection for metastatic colorectal cancer. J Am Coll Surg 185:554-559
15. Minagawa M, Makuuchi M, Torzilli G et al (2000) Extension of the frontiers of surgical indications in the treatment of liver metastases from colorectal cancer. Long-term results. Ann Surg 231:487-499
16. Oussoultzoglou E, Romain B, Panaro F et al (2009) Long-term survival after liver resection for colorectal liver metastases in patients with hepatic pedicle lymph nodes involvement in the era of new chemotherapy regimens. Ann Surg 249:879-886
17. Elias D, Gilly F, Boutitie F et al (2010) Peritoneal colorectal carcinomatosis treated with surgery and perioperative intraperitoneal chemotherapy: retrospective analysis of 523 patients from a multicentric French study. J Clin Oncol 28:63-68

18. Viganò L, Capussotti L, Laurent C et al (2010) Is progression while on neoadjuvant chemotherapy always a contraindication to liver resection for colorectal metastases? HPB 12S1:109-110
19. Neumann UP, Thelen A, Rocken C et al (2009) Nonresponse to pre-operative chemotherapy does not preclude long-term survival after liver resection in patients with colorectal liver metastases. Surgery 146:52-59
20. Kishi Y, Abdalla EK, Chun YS et al (2009) Three hundred and one consecutive extended right hepatectomies. Evaluation of outcome based on systematic liver volumetry. Ann Surg 250:540-548
21. Ferrero A, Viganò L, Polastri R et al (2007) Postoperative liver dysfunction and future remnant liver where is the limit? Results of a prospective study. World J Surg 31:1643-1651
22. Charnsangavej C, Clary B, Fong Y et al (2006) Selection of patients for resection of hepatic colorectal metastases: expert consensus statement. Ann Surg Oncol 13:1261-1268
23. Elias D, Cavalcanti A, Sabourin JC et al (1998) Results of 136 curative hepatectomies with a safety margin of less than 10 mm for colorectal metastases. J Surg Oncol 69:88-93
24. Adam R, Delvart V, Pascal G, et al (2004) Rescue surgey for unresectable colorectal liver metastases downstaged by chemotherapy. A model to predict long-term survival. Ann Surg 240:644-658
25. Charnsangavej C, Clary B, Fong Y et al (2006) Selection of patients for resection of hepatic colorectal metastases: expert consensus statement. Ann Surg Oncol 13:1261-1268
26. Are C, Gonen M, Zazzali K et al (2007) The impact of margins on outcome after hepatic resection for colorectal metastases. Ann Surg 246:295-300
27. Konopke R, Kersting S, Makowiec F et al (2008) Resection of colorectal liver metastases: is a resection margin of 3 mm enough? World J Surg 32:2047-2056
28. Nuzzo G, Giuliante F, Ardito F et al (2008) Influence of surgical margin on type of recurrence after liver resection for colorectal metastases: a single-center experience. Surgery 143:384-393
29. Muratore A, Ribero D, Zimmitti G et al (2010) Resection margin and recurrence-free survival after liver resection of colorectal metastases. Ann Surg Oncol 17:1324-1329

Surgical Strategy

4

Abstract Surgical strategy is the key to successful treatment of patients with colorectal liver metastases. The use of intraoperative ultrasonography has become mandatory at the beginning of the operation, as it allows better staging of the disease but also during every step of the resection, guiding the hepatectomy such that it is safer and easier. Intraoperative ultrasonography makes parenchyma-sparing resections possible, improving the likelihood of better preserved postoperative liver function, decreasing the risk of liver dysfunction, and facilitating re-resection in case of hepatic recurrences. The role of laparoscopic resection is still debated, but its potential advantages include the fact that it offers a minimally invasive approach for selected patients with limited disease. Pedicle clamping is often used during resection to decrease intraoperative blood loss; its impact on outcome in patients with colorectal metastases is discussed herein.

4.1
Introduction

The surgical technique of hepatectomy for colorectal liver metastases does not differ from that used for other primary or metastatic tumors of the liver. Nevertheless, surgical strategy is patient-dependent in particular cases and the type of resection should be tailored accordingly. We strongly recommend the routine use of intraoperative ultrasonography (IOUS) not only for disease staging at the beginning of the operation, but also during every step of the resection. By guiding the hepatectomy, IOUS makes the procedure safer and easier. IOUS also allows for parenchyma-sparing resections, thus improving the likelihood of better preserved postoperative liver function, decreasing the risk of liver dysfunction, and facilitating re-resection in patients with hepatic recurrences. The role of laparoscopic resections and the impact of pedicle clamping during hepatectomy on the outcome of patients with colorectal metastases are discussed herein.

A. Ferrero (✉)
Division of Hepato-Bilio-Pancreatic and Digestive Surgery, Mauriziano "Umberto I" Hospital, Turin, Italy

Surgical Treatment of Colorectal Liver Metastases. Lorenzo Capussotti (Ed.)
© Springer-Verlag Italia 2011

4.2
Intraoperative Ultrasonography

The first IOUS exploration of the liver was reported by Makuuchi in 1977. Since then it has been widely used in liver surgery and is nowadays an indispensable tool in the staging of neoplastic disease, in operative decision-making, and in surgical guidance during liver resection. Indeed, IOUS has several roles during liver surgery. It is the only way to precisely understand the liver's anatomy and to recognize vasculobiliary anomalies, which are very frequently encountered during hepatectomies. Intraoperatively, it allows staging of the disease, identifying the exact site of the lesion as well as new nodules that may have appeared within the liver. Moreover, it is useful during each step of the resection, guiding parenchymal transection and ligature of the Glissonian pedicles and veins. The use of IOUS to monitor blood flow during and after resection and to guide interstitial treatments associated with hepatectomy provides the surgeon with further operative advantages.

To adequately explore the liver, a medium- to top-level machine with dedicated intraoperative probes (T-shaped, finger-grip, or micro-Convex) is mandatory. The liver study is usually performed at 5 and 7.5 MHz. Use of ColorFlow and PowerFlow Imaging or the newest eFlow Imaging is essential in the evaluation of blood flow within the liver.

4.2.1
Technique

Ultrasound exploration of the liver can be done during laparotomy (IOUS) and laparoscopy (LUS). IOUS does not require wide incisions with complete exposure of the liver; rather, the use of dedicated probes allows satisfactory exploration through a limited incision, with easy access even to the virtual space between the liver dome and the diaphragm. An ultrasound study of the liver represents the first step in any form of hepatic surgery and does not require any previous mobilization, as a partial section of the falciform ligament facilitates exploration of the portal bifurcation and the caval confluence. The investigation is also simplified by gently pulling aside the sectioned round ligament. IOUS precedes any other maneuver involving the liver, as surgical dissection causes the spread of air into the anatomic planes, resulting in artifacts.

LUS is technically more demanding but is becoming increasingly popular, both for staging procedures and to guide laparoscopic liver resections. Laparoscopic probes have been recently developed with two to four movements and thus better adherence to the liver surface. We typically use two or three 10- to 12-mm trocars. The first trocar, for the 30° laparoscope, is inserted with an open technique in the umbilicus or close to it, according to previous abdominal scars. One or two trocars for the probe are then inserted in the right and left upper quadrants, along the planned laparotomy incision. The round and falciform ligaments are not sectioned but the adhesion is lysed to allow adequate access to both hemi-livers.

In IOUS and LUS, two standardized explorations are performed: the first assesses the anatomy of the liver (caval confluence, portal bifurcation, left segmental pedicles, right segmental pedicles, and hepatic pedicle), and the second the liver parenchyma and its lesions.

4.2.2
Ultrasonographic Characteristics of Colorectal Liver Metastases

Colorectal liver metastases show varied echogenicity on IOUS, appearing hypoechoic (Fig. 4.1), isoechoic (Fig. 4.2), or hyperechoic (Fig 4.3) compared to the surrounding liver tissue but depending on patient-specific (age, presence of liver disease, history of chemotherapy) and tumor-specific (size, location) factors. In a recent study by Choti et al. [1], the ultrasonographic appearance of colorectal liver metastasis was hypoechoic in 52.0%, isoechoic in 35.7%, and hyperechoic in 12.3% of cases. Such information is important because it may be used to predict the IOUS appearance of otherwise occult lesions. After the patient has received chemotherapy, it is not unusual to find hyperechoic spots with a posterior shadow within the lesions, caused by tumor necrosis (Fig. 4.4). The echogenicity of the metastasis can influence the surgeon's ability to detect lesions on IOUS, because isoechoic lesions may be more difficult to discriminate from the adjacent liver parenchyma. Sometimes an isoechoic metastasis can be visualized by looking for an indirect sign, such as compression of a vessel or bile duct dilatation (Fig. 4.5a, b). In such cases, contrast-enhanced IOUS (CE-IOUS) can provide more information. Colorectal liver metastases have a hypovascular appearance in the arterial phase, with possible peripheral rim-like enhancement, but are hypovascular in the portal-venous and late phases (Fig. 4.6). The echogenic appearance of colorectal metastases has been reported to be an independent prognostic factor of survival after curative hepatic resection. In particular, patients with hypoechoic hepatic metastases on IOUS were

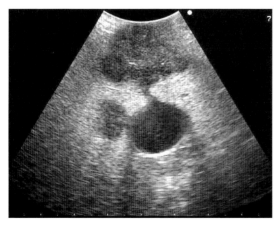

Fig. 4.1 Hypoechoic colorectal metastasis in Sg1 infiltrating a short hepatic vein

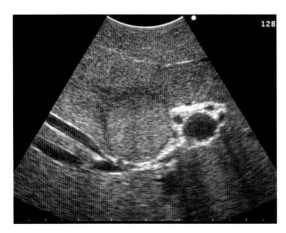

Fig. 4.2 Isoechoic colorectal metastasis between anterior and posterior right portal pedicles

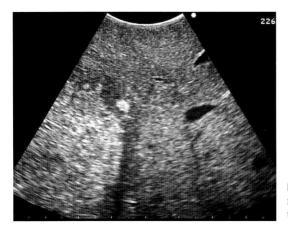

Fig. 4.3 Hyperechoic colorectal metastasis in Sg8 with satellite nodule

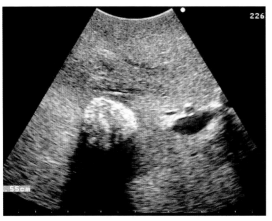

Fig. 4.4 Colorectal metastasis after neoadjuvant chemotherapy: hyperechoic spots with a posterior shadow, caused by tumor necrosis

4 Surgical Strategy

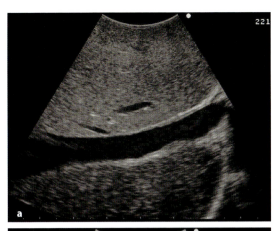

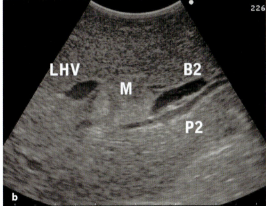

Fig. 4.5 Indirect signs of isoechoic colorectal metastases. **a** Loss of hyperechoic layer of the right hepatic vein wall caused by tumor infiltration; **b** segmental bile duct dilatation caused by tumor infiltration. *B2*, Sg2 bile duct; *LHV*, left hepatic vein; *M*, Metastasis; *P2*, Sg2 portal branch

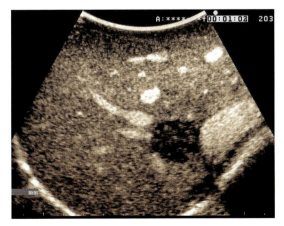

Fig. 4.6 Contrast-enhanced intraoperative ultrasonography (CE-IOUS), portal phase: colorectal metastasis infiltrating the right hepatic vein

at significantly higher risk of disease-specific death and had a significantly shorter median survival [2].

4.2.3
Intraoperative Staging

IOUS is an important tool for accurate staging of colorectal liver metastases at the time of resection. Even after careful preoperative imaging, new intraoperative findings or findings different than those suggested on preoperative imaging studies are commonly detected using IOUS. During surgery, IOUS is associated with the highest sensitivity (95–99%) and specificity (95–100%) concerning the number and localization of hepatic lesions and their relation with major vascular and biliary structures [3, 4]. Specifically, IOUS has been reported to identify at least one additional malignant lesion in 10–12% of patients. Furthermore, in 20% of patients with colorectal metastases, IOUS offers new information that alters the operative plan [5]. Preoperative imaging usually misses liver metastases, depending on their size and site. Preoperative CT scan significantly misses more lesions in Sg3 and Sg4, adjacent to the falciform ligament, or on the surface of the liver [6]. Only a few series have examined the additive value of CE-IOUS, reporting the identification of additional colorectal liver metastases in 13–19% of patients [7, 8]. The future availability of new contrast agents, such as sonazoid, a microbubble agent that provides a parenchyma-specific contrast image based on its accumulation in Kupffer cells, will probably enhance the yield of IOUS in detecting new lesions [9].

To reveal unresectable disease not detected on radiological imaging, routine use of laparoscopy before liver resection has been advocated. Laparoscopic exploration can easily visualize peritoneal carcinomatosis or advanced nodal disease, both of which can preclude curative resection. The addition of LUS enables staging laparoscopy to visualize incurable disease not detected by radiological imaging in up to 58% of patients [10]. Nevertheless, laparoscopy seems to have a low diagnostic yield in patients without adverse prognostic factors [11] and should probably be used only in selected patients at high risk of new pathological findings. LUS can guide the biopsy of new liver nodules potentially representing metastasis or adenopathy.

4.2.4
IOUS and Liver Resection

The constant use of the IOUS by the surgeon him/herself during the operation is considered nowadays mandatory, in order to guide the resection and to make it safer and easier. After the exploration of the liver in order to better stage the disease, IOUS can precisely detect the relationships between the lesion and the vascular structures. Hepatic vein infiltration can be visualized when the hyperechoic rim of the venous wall is interrupted by tumor (Fig. 4.7). Infiltration of a segmental or subsegmental portal pedicle should always be suspected when biliary dilatation is associated with

4 Surgical Strategy

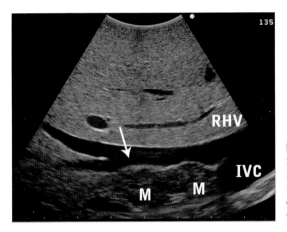

Fig. 4.7 Two adjacent colorectal metastases in Sg7 infiltrating the right hepatic vein (*RHV*). *IVC*, inferior vena cava; *M*, Metastasis. The *arrow* shows a loss of the hyperechoic layer of the RHV wall

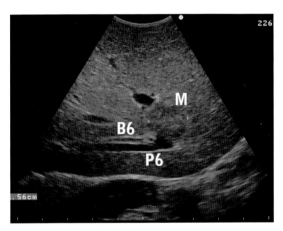

Fig. 4.8 Colorectal metastasis infiltrating Sg6 Glissonian pedicle with segmental bile duct dilatation. *B6*, Sg6 bile duct; *M*, Metastasis; *P6*, Sg6 portal branch

adhesion of the tumor (Fig. 4.8). If vascular infiltration is suspected, the vessel should be ligated and sectioned in order to allow radical resection. Otherwise, the lesion can be dissected from the vessel, even if a thin surgical margin is obtained [12]. When a major hepatic vein is infiltrated by tumor and is to be ligated, it may not be necessary to remove all of the liver parenchyma drained by that vein. This is the case in bisegmentectomy Sg7-8 for a metastasis infiltrating the right hepatic vein (RHV), which is possible in the presence of an inferior right hepatic vein draining Sg6 [13, 14]. In the absence of an inferior RHV, flow in the Sg6 portal pedicle should be evaluated before and after RHV clamping: if color-Doppler IOUS shows that portal flow in Sg6 remains hepatopetal, a bisegmentectomy Sg7-8 with ligation of the RHV can be performed without any congestion of the remaining Sg6 (Fig. 4.9). This is possible due to the patency of anastomotic branches between the right and middle hepatic veins [14]. When color-Doppler shows an inverted flow in the posterior portal pedicle, a right hepatectomy should be performed (Fig. 4.10). These detailed new

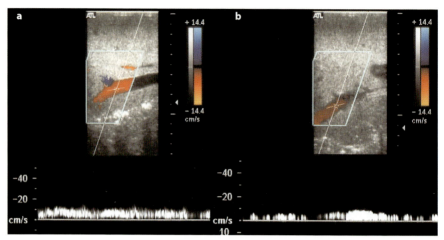

Fig. 4.9 Flow in the Sg6 portal branch in a patient with colorectal metastasis infiltrating the right hepatic vein in the absence of the inferior right hepatic vein. **a** Before right hepatic vein clamping; **b** after right hepatic vein clamping: flow is reduced, but still hepatopetal

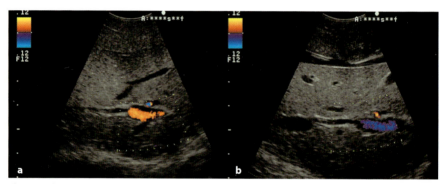

Fig. 4.10 Flow in the Sg6 portal branch in a patient with colorectal metastasis infiltrating the right hepatic vein in the absence of the inferior right hepatic vein. **a** Before right hepatic vein clamping; **b** after right hepatic vein clamping: flow is inverted. The patient underwent right hepatectomy

findings may lead to modifications of the intraoperative strategy, such that the type of resection is usually decided at the end of the IOUS study.

During parenchymal transection, IOUS allows monitoring of the correct surgical plane in order to maintain an adequate surgical margin and avoid lesions to major vascular structures. The transection plane is easily recognized as a hyperechoic layer with distal artifacts (Fig. 4.11). During the transection, when a vessel is encountered and is to be ligated, IOUS allows a correct understanding of the anatomy, which is confirmed using the "hooking technique:" the surgeon tapes the vessel and pulls it, under ultrasound exploration, to visualize the exact branch to be sectioned [15]. At the end of the operation, the raw cut surface of the liver can be visualized by IOUS,

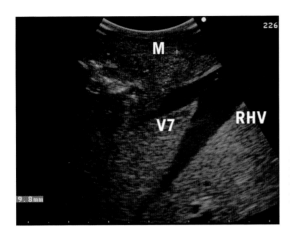

Fig. 4.11 Atypical resection of Sg7. IOUS shows the correct transection plane, sparing the right hepatic vein. *M*, Metastasis; *RHV,* right hepatic vein; *V7,* branch of the right hepatic vein from Sg7

allowing the detection of any remaining lesion. The specimen itself can be explored outside the operative field to check the lesions and the surgical margin.

4.3
Parenchyma-sparing Surgery

The goal of sparing healthy liver parenchyma by performing a limited resection instead of a major hepatectomy for colorectal liver metastases is becoming widely accepted [16-18] and is supported by pathological, oncological, and technical findings. Intrahepatic micrometastases via the portal branch are uncommon in case of colorectal liver metastases, as reported by Yamamoto et al. in a histopathological study [19]; when satellitosis occurs, tumor deposits are usually encountered within 2 mm from the border of the main nodule [20]. As already reported in Chap. 3 of this volume, recent studies have demonstrated that the width of a negative surgical margin does not affect either the risk of recurrence or overall survival. Based on their design, conservative operations are more likely to be associated with close margins: a limited resection with a negative margin is easily obtained when the nodule is superficial, but could be difficult if the metastasis is sited deeply within the liver. The increased use of IOUS is crucial for this kind of surgery as it easily identifies the site and the number of lesions, showing the exact relationships between the tumor and the main vascular structures. Moreover, IOUS is useful to check the correct plane during parenchymal transection. The choice of the type of hepatectomy should be individualized for each patient, according to the size, number, and location of the metastases.

The aim of parenchyma-sparing strategy is to permit resection of all metastases, with negative histologic margins, while preserving as much functional hepatic parenchyma as possible. In such cases, postoperative liver function is well preserved in patients who have undergone both wedge resection [21] (Fig 4.12) and anatomic bisegmentectomy as an alternative to major hepatectomy [22] (Fig. 4.13).

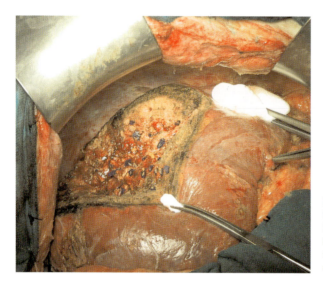

Fig. 4.12 Large atypical resection of segment 8, extending to segments 5 and 7, for a metachronous 5.6-cm metastasis infiltrating the origin of P8

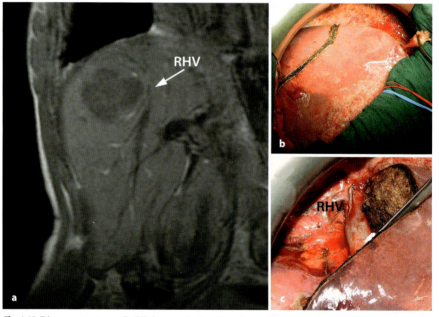

Fig. 4.13 Bisegmentectomy Sg7/8 in a patient with a 5-cm liver metastases infiltrating the right hepatic vein (*RHV*) close to the hepato-caval confluence. Intraoperative color-Doppler analysis showed sufficient venous drainage after RHV clamping. **a** MRI shows the vascular relationship of the tumor. **b** Transection line drawn on the liver surface. **c** Raw cut surface at the end of the parenchymal transection with the ligated RHV

We recently showed that, in the postoperative course, the serum bilirubin level was significantly lower and prothrombin time significantly higher in patients treated by more conservative procedures. Moreover, three patients out of 36 who underwent right hepatectomy experienced liver dysfunction in the postoperative course, while no liver dysfunction occurred in the control group [22]. These results concerning liver function are even more interesting if we consider the adverse effects of neoadjuvant chemotherapy on the liver parenchyma.

Another advantage of leaving the maximal amount of liver parenchyma is to improve the possibility of repeat hepatectomy in case of liver recurrence. Further on, we will discuss the observation that patients who undergo a second or third liver resection for recurrent liver metastases may have longer survival. The greater the number of major vascular structures that are preserved within the liver during the first hepatectomy, the higher the number of patients who will benefit from a second and possibly a third liver resection in case of parenchymal relapse.

Conservative bisegmentectomy in case of metastases sited deeply within the liver can result in narrow surgical margins, with the risk of exposing the tumor during the parenchymal transection. The intensive use of IOUS during hepatectomy can decrease this risk, but unfortunately cannot avoid it. In our series, both surgical margin width and non-radical resections were similar in the two groups. The overall recurrence rates were similar too. The long-term results of our series demonstrated that the type of hepatectomy, whether a right hepatectomy or a bisegmentectomy, does not influence recurrence-free and overall survival rates [22].

In conclusion, parenchyma-sparing liver resection is a safe alternative to major hepatectomy in patients with colorectal liver metastases, provided that a radical intervention is performed. This approach better preserves postoperative liver function, decreasing the risk of liver dysfunction, and yields similar survival results as well as an improved opportunity to re-resect hepatic recurrences.

4.4
Laparoscopic Liver Resection

Almost 3000 laparoscopic liver resections (LLRs) [23] have been performed worldwide since 1992, when Gagner [24] carried out the first non-anatomic resection of a liver tumor. Of the patients who underwent resection, 50% suffered from malignant tumors, with colorectal liver metastases in 35% of this group [23]. Some authors have pointed out the advantages of LLR, such as small incisions with preservation of the abdominal wall, less postoperative pain, and shorter hospital stays [25]. However, LLR is technically demanding, requiring considerable experience in both hepatobiliary surgery and advanced laparoscopic surgery as well as the availability of appropriate technology [23]. A recent study [26] reported that the learning curve of LLR was similar to that of laparoscopic colonic surgery. Finally, it has also been suggested that IOUS is inadequate to assess additional or small liver lesions during LLR [27]. The most favorable indication for LLR is a solitary lesion, ≤ 5 cm, located on

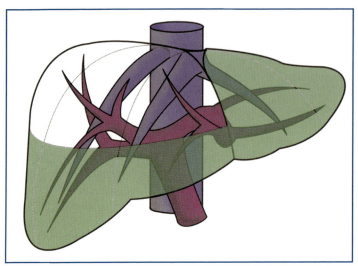

Fig. 4.14 Laparoscopic segments

left lateral (Sg2-3) and anterior right (Sg5-6) segments (Fig. 4.14). Patients with tumors > 5 cm that are central, multiple, bilateral, or have connections with the liver hilum, major hepatic veins, or the inferior vena cava are currently not considered to be the best candidates for a laparoscopic approach [23]. Nevertheless, in some centers, even these lesions are addressed laparoscopically [24].

4.4.1
Feasibility and Safety

The feasibility and safety of LLR have been demonstrated in several reports [28, 29]. In a recent review of 127 published papers on minimally invasive hepatic resections, nine postoperative deaths were reported after 2804 LLRs (0.3% mortality). No intraoperative deaths have been reported. The complication rate was 10.5%, ranging from 0% to 50% [23]. Bile leak was the most common liver-related postoperative complication. Nevertheless, the incidence of 42 bile leaks (1.5%) is similar to that reported in the majority of open resection series. Other liver-related complications included transient liver failure/ascites (1%) and liver abscess. Complications tended to occur more frequently after LLR for hepatocellular carcinoma (50%) than after the procedure was performed for colorectal metastases (11%) ($p = 0.02$), most likely due to the underlying liver disease, with the potential for postoperative liver failure [30]. Koffron et al. [31] provided the largest single-center experience in LLR, with 300 procedures performed from July 2001 to November 2006. These were compared with 100 contemporaneous open liver resections in patients matched for age, type of resection, benign vs. malignant tumor origin, and presence of liver cirrhosis. Compared with the open resection group, the laparoscopic resection group fared better in operative time (99 vs. 182 min), blood loss (102 vs. 325 ml), transfusion requirement (0.007% vs. 0.08%), length of stay (1.9 vs. 5.4 days), and overall operative complications (9.3% vs. 22%).

Although the laparoscopic cases certainly entailed patient selection bias (compared with open hepatic surgery), these reported cases provide evidence that the mortality and morbidity of LLR do not exceed that of open resection. The overall conversion rate of 4.1% to an open procedure in the collective series (116 of 2804 cases) should not be deemed as failure, and conversion to open resection should be expedited if bleeding cannot be controlled laparoscopically, adequate resection margins cannot be obtained, or adhesions preclude laparoscopic progress [23]. Almost 80% of procedures are converted to open surgery due to hemorrhage [32] but if managed by an expert surgeon this does not worsen outcome. Hand assistance can be useful in selected cases to avoid conversion [33].

4.4.2
Oncological Results

When laparoscopic liver resection is performed for cancer, there must be no compromise in the oncological integrity of the operation. Negative margins should always be the goal. Early attempts at laparoscopic resection of cancers were associated with high numbers of abdominal metastases, especially at port sites, but also in the peritoneal cavity [34]. More recent prospective studies in which proper oncological surgery ("no touch" technique, specimen bag, and abdominal wall protection) was ensured do not seem to confirm this trend [35].

Particular care should be taken during limited resections in anterior segments (segments 4 and 5), where the posterior margin may be more difficult to assess. Bryant et al. [37] proposed radiofrequency pre-coagulation as a useful technique to increase margins in some marginal limited resections, but there are few reports indicating that radiofrequency ablation can reduce the risk of margin recurrence.

Few survival data for colorectal liver metastases have been published [38-40]. Vibert et al. [38] reported on 41 LLRs for colorectal cancer, with overall survival rates at 1 year and 3 years of 97% and 87%, respectively. Disease-free survivals at 1 year and 3 years were 74% and 51%, respectively. No port-site metastases were noted during the follow-up period. A recent retrospective study [40] compared long-term results of liver resection for colorectal metastases performed laparoscopically vs. by an open procedure. Patients were treated in two centers, one specialized in LLR and the other in open hepatectomies, and compared on an intention to treat basis using nine preoperative prognostic criteria. For LLR, 1-, 3-, and 5-year patient survival was 97%, 82%, and 64%, respectively, while in the open group the corresponding rates were 97%, 70%, and 56%, respectively. Regarding disease-free survival, the 1-, 3-, and 5-year rates were 70%, 47%, and 35% for the LLR group and 70%, 40%, and 27 for the open group, respectively.

No randomized clinical trial comparing laparoscopic with open hepatic resection for cancer has been conducted. Impediments to this type of trial include the large number of patients required, the variability of techniques among surgeons, and the resistance of patients to potentially being randomized to a more invasive procedure.

In conclusion, the safety and feasibility of LLR in selected patients merit a place for this technique in the armamentarium of the liver surgeon. For LLR to be effective, specific training and access to adequate technology are required. Patient selection must be accurate. Further prospective evaluation will allow assessment of the results of laparoscopy in the treatment of liver colorectal metastases.

4.5
Hepatic Pedicle Clamping

Liver resection is still associated with a high risk of major intraoperative blood loss and perioperative blood transfusion, even with the improvements in surgical and anesthetic techniques [41]. Several studies have suggested that perioperative blood loss and transfusions are negative prognostic factors with respect to postoperative outcome, tumor recurrence, and long-term survival [42]. Strategies to minimize blood loss during transection of the hepatic parenchyma include vascular inflow occlusion. Nevertheless, the liver poorly tolerates prolonged periods of ischemia, which results in irreversible damage (ischemia/reperfusion damage) [43, 44]. To address the issue of ischemia–reperfusion injury, intermittent portal triad clamping (PTC), ischemic pre-conditioning, and selective clamping have been proposed as modifications of the original Pringle maneuver.

4.5.1
Strategies To Reduce Reperfusion Injuries

Several strategies have been devised to reduce reperfusion injury (pharmacological interventions) or to increase the ischemic tolerance of the liver (ischemic pre-conditioning, intermittent PTC, selective clamping).

Pharmacological interventions. In a recent review [45], five randomized trials evaluating nine different pharmacological interventions were analyzed. There were no significant differences between the groups in terms of mortality, liver failure, or postoperative complications. Our randomized study, published in 2003, confirmed that preoperative steroid administration does not improve short-term outcome [46] .

Ischemic preconditioning. A review published in 2009 [47] examined four randomized clinical trials in which a total of 271 patients were randomized to ischemic pre-conditioning ($n = 135$) or no ischemic preconditioning ($n = 136$) prior to continuous vascular occlusion. In spite of lower enzyme markers of liver injury in the ischemic preconditioning group, there was no difference in mortality, liver function, or other morbidity between the two groups. The same study [47] reported a reduction in the blood transfusion requirements in the ischemic preconditioning group, but there was no difference in blood loss between the two groups.

Intermittent Pringle maneuver. A randomized clinical study by Belghiti et al. [48] examining patients undergoing liver resection showed that intermittent clamping using multiple cycles of 15 min of ischemia and 5 min of reperfusion was associated with decreased injury compared with similar periods of continuous inflow occlusion. Three studies compared intermittent PTC with no hepatic inflow occlusion; a meta-analysis [49] of these trials showed no difference in postoperative overall morbidity or mortality between patients undergoing intermittent PTC or no PTC. In contrast to the study by Chouker et al. [50], in which there was significantly less blood loss with continuous PTC than in patients not treated by PTC, our study [51] showed that patients with intermittent PTC had a similar amount of blood loss as those without PTC.

Selective clamping. Portal vein and artery dissection to perform selective clamping is time consuming, and previous comparisons by means of retrospective [52, 53] and randomized [54] studies did not show any difference in the postoperative outcome.

In conclusion, current evidence shows no benefit for PTC on outcome after liver resection. Although early studies reported significantly reduced blood loss with PTC, more recent studies have not confirmed this finding. As reported in our study [51], any type of liver resection can be performed safely without pedicle clamping. This is due to advances in hepatic surgery, which now permit resections with limited blood loss, even without hepatic inflow occlusion. Safe liver surgery requires knowledge of the standard techniques of vascular occlusion for "on demand" use when necessary to reduce blood loss.

4.5.2
Impact of Hepatic Pedicle Clamping on Long-term Outcome

A recent experimental study found that prolonged vascular clamping (> 45 min) may induce a five- or six-fold local acceleration of tumor growth [55]. The same authors subsequently demonstrated that the safe upper limit of vascular clamping is 20 min [56]. Only a few reports have focused on the impact of pedicle clamping on long-term outcome [57, 58]. Wong et al. [58] recently reported a large series of patients who underwent hepatic resection for colorectal metastases: 289 with intermittent Pringle maneuver and 274 without. They found that the Pringle maneuver was not associated with worse long-term outcome; however, the the two groups were not compared in a randomized setting. Our recent prospective study [59] evaluated the impact of pedicle clamping on survival outcomes; we analyzed long-term results, prospectively collected, of 80 patients with colorectal liver metastases randomized in the previous study to undergo hepatectomy with (39 patients) or without (41 patients) pedicle clamping. Overall disease-free survival rates at 1-, 3-, and 5-years were similar between the two groups. Survival rates of a subset of patients who underwent hepatectomy with a Pringle maneuver time > 45 min were compared with those of patients who were operated on without PTC. Also in this case, the overall and disease-free survival rates were similar. In a murine model [56] of steatotic liver, the outgrowth of micrometastases after pedicle clamping was significantly higher than in healthy livers. In our study, even considering patients with liver steatosis, no significant differences of overall and disease-free survival were found in the two groups.

In conclusion, pedicle clamping does not seem to affect survival after liver resection in patients with colorectal liver metastases, but a randomized clinical trial is needed to confirm these results.

References

1. Choti MA, Kaloma F, de Oliveira ML et al (2008) Patient variability in intraoperative ultrasonographic characteristics of colorectal liver metastases. Arch Surg 143:29-34
2. DeOliveira ML, Pawlik TM, Gleisner AL et al (2007) Echogenic appearance of colorectal liver metastases on intraoperative ultrasonography is associated with survival after hepatic resection. J Gastrointest Surg 11:970-6
3. Bhattacharjya S, Bhattacharjya T, Baber S et al (2004) Prospective study of contrast-enhanced computed tomography, computed tomography during arterioportography, and magnetic resonance imaging for staging colorectal liver metastases for liver resection. Br J Surg 91:1361-9
4. Schmidt J, Strotzer M, Fraunhofer S et al (2000) Intraoperative ultrasonography versus helical computed tomography and computed tomography with arterioportography in diagnosing colorectal liver metastases: lesion-by-lesion analysis. World J Surg 24:43-7
5. Zacherl J, Scheuba C, Imhof M et al (2002) Current value of intraoperative sonography during surgery for hepatic neoplasms. World J Surg 26:550-554
6. Foroutani A, Garland AM, Berber E et al (2000) Laparoscopic ultrasound vs triphasic computed tomography for detecting liver tumors. Arch Surg 135:933-8
7. Torzilli G, Del Fabbro D, Palmisano A et al (2005) Contrast-enhanced intraoperative ultrasonography during hepatectomies for colorectal cancer liver metastases. J Gastrointest Surg 9:1148-53
8. Leen E, Ceccotti P, Moug SJ et al (2006) Potential value of contrast-enhanced intraoperative ultrasonography during partial hepatectomy for metastases: an essential investigation before resection? Ann Surg 243:236-40
9. Nakano H, Ishida Y, Hatakeyama T et al (2008) Contrast-enhanced intraoperative ultrasonography equipped with late Kupffer-phase image obtained by sonazoid in patients with colorectal liver metastases. World J Gastroenterol 14:3207-3211
10. Mann CD, Neal CP, Metcalfe MS et al (2007) Clinical Risk Score predicts yield of staging laparoscopy in patients with colorectal liver metastases. Br J Surg 94(7):855-9
11. Jarnagin WR, Conlon K, Bodniewicz J et al (2001) A clinical scoring system predicts the yield of diagnostic laparoscopy in patients with potentially resectable hepatic colorectal metastases. Cancer 91:1121-28
12. Torzilli G, Montorsi M, Donadon M et al (2005) "Radical but conservative" is the main goal for ultrasonography-guided liver resection: prospective validation of this approach. J Am Coll Surg 201:517-28
13. Makuuchi M, Hasegawa H, Yamazaki S et al (1987) Four new hepatectomy procedures for resection of the right hepatic vein and preservation of the inferior right hepatic vein. Surg Gynecol Obstet 164:68-72

14. Capussotti L, Ferrero A, Viganò L et al (2006) Hepatic bisegmentectomy 7-8 for a colorectal metastasis. Eur J Surg Oncol 32:469-71
15. Torzilli G, Montorsi M, Gambetti A et al (2005) Utility of the hooking technique for cases of major hepatectomy. Surg Endosc 19:1156-7
16. Chouillard E, Cherqui D, Tayar C et al (2003) Anatomical bi- and trisegmentectomies as alternatives to extensive liver resections. Ann Surg 238(1):29-34
17. Kokudo N, Tada K, Seki M et al (2001) Anatomical major resection versus nonanatomical limited resection for liver metastases from colorectal carcinoma. Am J Surg 181:153-159
18. Muratore A, Conti P, Amisano M et al (2005) Bisegmentectomy 7-8 as alternative to more extensive liver resections. J Am Coll Surg 200:224-228
19. Yamamoto J, Sugihara K, Kosuge T et al (1995) Pathologic support for limited hepatectomy in the treatment of liver metastases from colorectal cancer. Ann Surg 221:74-78
20. Kokudo N, Miki Y, Sugai S et al (2002) Genetic and histological assessment of surgical margins in resected liver metastases from colorectal carcinoma: minimum surgical margins for successful resection. Arch Surg 137:833-840
21. Zorzi D, Mullen JT, Abdalla EK et al (2006) Comparison between hepatic wedge resection and anatomic resection for colorectal liver metastases. J Gastrointest Surg 10:86-94
22. Ferrero A, Viganò L, Lo Tesoriere R et al (2009) Bisegmentectomies as alternative to right hepatectomy in the treatment of colorectal liver metastases. Hepatogastroenterology 56:1429-35
23. KT Nguyen, TC Gamblin, Geller DA (2009) World Review of Laparoscopic Liver Resection–2,804 Patients. Ann Surg 250:831-841
24. Gayet B, Cavaliere D, Vibert E et al (2007) Totally laparoscopic right hepatectomy Am J Surg 194:685–689
25. Cherqui D, Husson E, Hammoud R et al (2000) Laparoscopic liver resections: a feasibility study in 30 patients. Ann Surg 232:753–762
26. Viganò L, Laurent A, Tayar C et al (2009) The learning curve in laparoscopic liver resection: improved feasibility and reproducibility. Ann Surg 250:772-782
27. Laurent A, Cherqui D, Lesurtel M et al (2003) Laparoscopic liver resection for subcapsular hepatocellular carcinoma complicating chronic liver disease. Arch Surg 138:763–769
28. Buell JF, Cherqui D, Geller DA et al (2009) The International Position on Laparoscopic Liver Surgery: The Louisville Statement, 2008 Ann Surg 250:825-30
29. Cherqui D, Husson E, Hammoud R et al (2000) Laparoscopic liver resections: a feasibility study in 30 patients. Ann Surg 232:753-762
30. Gigot JF, Glineur D, Santiago Azagra J et al (2002) Hepatobiliary and Pancreatic Section of the Royal Belgian Society of Surgery and the Belgian Group for Endoscopic Surgery: Laparoscopic liver resection for malignant liver tumors: preliminary results of a multicenter European study Ann Surg 236:90-97
31. Koffron AJ, Auffenberg G, Kung R et al (2007) Evaluation of 300 minimally invasive liver resections at a single institution: less is more. Ann Surg 246:385-392
32. Gigot JF, Glineur D, Santiago Azagra J et al (2002) Laparoscopic liver resection for malignant liver tumors: preliminary results of a multicenter European study. Ann Surg 236:90-97
33. Viganò L, Tayar C, Laurent A, Cherqui D (2009) Laparoscopic liver resection: a systematic review. J Hepatobiliary Pancreat Surg. 16:410-421
34. Johnstone PAS, Rohde DC, Swartz Se et al (1996) Portsite recurrences after laparoscopic and thoracoscopic procedures in malignacy. J Clin Oncol 14:1950-1956
35. Poulin EC, Mamazza J, Schlachta C et al (1995) Laparoscopic resection does not adversely affect early survival curves in patients undergoing surgery for colorectal adenocarcinoma. Ann Surg 229:487-492
36. Bryant R, Laurent A, Tayar C et al (2009) Laparoscopic Liver Resection–Understanding its Role in Current Practice The Henri Mondor Hospital Experience Ann Surg 250:103-111

37. Hompes D, Aerts R, Penninckx F et al (2007) Laparoscopic liver resection using radiofrequency coagulation. Surg Endosc 21:175-180
38. Vibert E, Perniceni T, Levard H et al (2006) Laparoscopic liver resection. Br J Surg 93:67-72
39. Robles R, Marin C, Abellan B et al (2008) A new approach to hand-assisted laparoscopic liver surgery. Surg Endosc 22:2357-2364
40. Castaing D, Vibert E, Ricca L et al (2009) Oncologic Results of Laparoscopic Versus Open Hepatectomy for Colorectal Liver Metastases in Two Specialized Centers. Ann Surg 250: 849–855
41. Nagorney DM, van Heerden JA, Ilstrup DM et al (1989) Primary hepatic malignancy: surgical management and determinants of survival. Surgery 106:740-749
42. Kooby DA, Stockman J, Ben-Porat L et al (2003) Influence of transfusion on perioperative and lomg-term outcome in patients following hepatic resection for colorectal metastasis. Ann Surg 237:860-869
43. Yin XY, Lai PBS, Lee JFY et al (2000) Effects of hepatic blood inflow occlusion on liver regeneration following partial hepatectomy in an experimental model of cirrhosis. Br J Surg 87:1510–1515
44. Teoh NC, Farrell GC (2003) Hepatic ischemia reperfusion injury: pathogenic mechanisms and basis for hepatoprotection. J Gastroenterol Hepatol 18:891-902
45. Abu-Amara M, Gurusamy KS, Glantzounis G et al (2009) Pharmacological interventions for ischaemia reperfusion injury in liver resection surgery performed under vascular control. Cochrane Database Syst Rev (4). Art No CD008154
46. Muratore A, Ribero D, Ferrero A et al (2003) Prospective randomized study of steroids in the prevention of ischaemic injury during hepatic resection with pedicle clamping. Br J Surg 90:17-22
47. Gurusamy KS, Kumar Y, Pamecha V et al (2009) Ischaemic pre-conditioning for elective liver resections performed under vascular occlusion. Cochrane Database Syst Rev (1). Art No CD007629
48. Belghiti J, Noun R, Malafosse R et al (1999) Continuous versus intermittent portal triad clamping for liver resection. Ann Surg 229:369-375
49. Rahbari NN, Wente MN, Schemmer P et al (2008) Systematic review and meta-analysis of the effect of portal triad clamping on outcome after hepatic resection. Br J Surg 95:424-32
50. Chouker A, Schachtner T, Schauer R et al (2004) Effects of Pringle manoeuvre and ischaemic preconditioning on haemodynamic stability in patients undergoing elective hepatectomy: a randomized trial. Br J Anaesth 93:204-211
51. Capussotti L, Muratore A, Ferrero A et al (2006) Randomized clinical trial of liver resection with and without hepatic pedicle clamping. Br J Surg 93:685-689
52. Gotoh M, Monden M, Sakon M et al (1994) Hilar lobar vascular occlusion for hepatic resection. J Am Coll Surg 178:6-10
53. Takayama T, Makuuchi M, Inoue K et al (1998) Selective and unselective clamping in cirrhotic liver. Hepato Gastroenterol 45:376-380
54. Wu C-C, Yeh D-C, Ho W-H et al (2002) Occlusion of hepatic blood inflow for complex central liver resections in cirrhotic patients. Arch Surg137:1369-1376
55. van der Bilt JD, Kranenburg O, Nijkamp MW et al (2005) Ischemia/reperfusion accelerates the outgrowth of hepatic micrometastases in a highly standardized murine model. Hepatology 42:165-175
56. van der Bilt JD, Kranenburg O, Borren A et al (2008) Ageing and hepatic steatosis exacerbate ischemia/reperfusion-accelerated outgrowth of colorectal micrometastases. Ann Surg Oncol 15:1392-1398

57. Buell JF, Koffron A, Yoshida A et al (2000) Is any method of vascular control superior in hepatic resection of metastatic cancers? Longmire clamping, pringle maneuver, and total vascular isolation. Arch Surg 136:569-575
58. Wong KH, Hamady ZZ, Malik HZ et al (2008) Intermittent Pringle manoeuvre is not associated with adverse long-term prognosis after resection for colorectal liver metastases. Br J Surg 95:985-989
59. Ferrero A, Russolillo N, Viganò L et al (2010) Does Pringle maneuver affect survival in patients with colorectal liver metastases? WJS in press

Results of Surgery and Prognostic Factors

5

Abstract Hepatic resection is the treatment of choice for colorectal liver metastases, with 5-year survival rates now approaching 60%. Postoperative morbidity and mortality are constantly decreasing. In particular, 90-day postoperative mortality has been reported in several series to be less than 1%. Several prognostic factors of poor outcome have been recognized but, at present, most of them cannot be used to select patients for resection. Future identification of molecular factors may aid in the prediction of prognosis and help to improve the selection of those patients most likely to benefit from surgery.

5.1
Introduction

Radical hepatic resection remains the only potentially curative therapy for patients with liver metastases from colorectal carcinoma. Over the past decades, improvements in patient selection, anesthesiologic monitoring, surgical techniques and perioperative critical care have resulted in a significant decrease in the surgical risk. A better understanding of the internal anatomy of the liver combined with the systematic use of intraoperative ultrasound has allowed for a precise mapping of the vascular structures as well as a clear definition of the extent of disease and the tumors' relationships, and thus for the optimal planning of surgical resections. Consequently, postoperative complications and mortality have been minimized. Likewise, long-term survival has been improved despite an increasingly aggressive surgical approach. In fact, larger, more complex procedures are now undertaken in patients with tumors once considered unresectable.

The purpose of this chapter is to review the results of hepatic resection in terms of short- and long-term outcomes, and to discuss the significance of various prognostic factors.

D. Ribero (✉)
Division of Hepato-Bilio-Pancreatic and Digestive Surgery, Mauriziano "Umberto I" Hospital, Turin, Italy

Surgical Treatment of Colorectal Liver Metastases. Lorenzo Capussotti (Ed.)
© Springer-Verlag Italia 2011

5.2
Short-term Results

Since the mid-1970s the mortality rate of hepatectomy has decreased from as high as 20% to less than 5% in recent series from high-volume centers. A systematic review of all published studies reporting short- and long-term results of surgical resection of colorectal liver metastases indicated a median mortality rate of 2.8% [1]. The most frequent cause of death was hepatic failure, in 18.4% of the cases, followed by postoperative hemorrhage (17.5%), generalized sepsis (16.5%), and cardiac failure (11.7%). Table 5.1 reports mortality rates in selected series from tertiary referral centers [2-18]. Notably, a mortality rate of < 1% has been confirmed. Recently, House et al. [16] compared the outcome of 1037 patients operated on between 1985 and 1998 with that of 563 patients who underwent resection between 1999 and 2004. Operative mortality significantly decreased from 2.5% in the first period to 1% in later years. Interestingly, the authors reported that when considering the 90-day mor-

Table 5.1 Perioperative mortality and morbidity of liver resection for colorectal metastases

Author	Year	Patients (*n*)	Major hepatectomy (%)	Morbidity (%)	Mortality (%)
Scheele [2]	1995	496	-	16	4.4
Nordliger [3]	1996	1568	64	23	2.3
Fong [4]	1999	1001	63	31	2.8
Minagawa [5]	2000	235	21	-	0
Choti [6]	2002	226	53	19	0.9
Ercolani [7]	2002	245	42	15	0.8
Adam [8]	2004	335	75	28	0.7
Fernandez [9]	2004	100	75	-	1
Jonas [10]	2007	660	66	27	2.5
Malik [11]	2007	700	65	29	3
Tomlinson [12]	2007	644	-	-	5
Are [13]	2007	1019	66	44	2
Rees [14]	2008	929	60	26	1.5[a]
Gold [15]	2008	440	84	29	5.4
House [16]	2010	1600	60	44	2[b]
Capussotti (unpublished)	2010	669	36	31	0.4

[a]Mortality was 1% in the most recent period (1999–2004; *n* of patients: 563)
[b]Included only multiple bilateral metastases

tality the number of deaths doubled compared to the number that would have been reported if the observational period had been limited to the traditional 30 postoperative days. This confirms the finding of Mullen et al. [21]. In their multicenter study, the results of 1059 non-cirrhotic patients who underwent major or extended hepatectomy at three major hepatobiliary institutions (University of Texas MD Anderson Cancer Center, Houston, TX; Duke University Medical Center, Durham, NC; and our institution), with 55.7% of the hepatectomies performed for colorectal metastases, were analyzed. The 30- and 90-day all-cause mortality rates were 3.2% and 4.7%, respectively, with a significant 47% increase in the postoperative mortality rate. Of these fatalities, 60% were related to hepatic failure, which remains the most relevant postoperative complication. In fact, in such circumstances patients often require prolonged stays in the intensive care unit, endure a protracted recovery, and can ultimately succumb to fatal hepatic failure. In the review by Simmonds et al. [1], hepatic failure, however, ranked sixth among the most common postoperative complications, after wound infection, generalized sepsis, pleural effusion, bile leak, and perihepatic abscess. Yet, to date, there is no standardized definition of postoperative hepatic insufficiency which might explain the wide range of frequencies (1–27%) with which this complication is reported to affect patient outcome. In addition, several postoperative complications, in particular infective ones, may cause sepsis and, as a consequence, hepatic insufficiency [22]. Overall, postoperative complication rates vary between 16% and 44% (Table 5.1). Reports indicate that several factors, including intraoperative blood loss and blood transfusion, a concomitant major extrahepatic procedure, comorbid medical conditions, and the number of resected segments, are independently associated with a greater likelihood of perioperative morbidity and mortality [21, 23]. In particular, the extent of resection appears to strongly influence the posthepatectomy incidence of adverse events. Jarnagin et al. [23] demonstrated in a large series of 1803 liver resections that operative mortality increased from < 1% in patients who underwent resection of < 3 segments to 5% and 7.8%, respectively, in those who had five or six segments resected. Similarly, in patients who underwent a resection of $\leq$ 1 segment, the complication rate was 32% while it increased progressively to 75% in patients who underwent resection of six segments. A similar trend was observed in our series consisting of 668 first resections for colorectal liver metastases, including 47 patients who underwent a two-stage hepatectomy, performed between January 1989 and December 2009. The overall morbidity rate was 30.9% and was significantly higher in patients undergoing major or extended resection (34.2%) than in patients treated with minor resection (26.2%). Two of the three patients who died within 90 days (mortality rate 0.4%) had undergone a major hepatic resection. Figure 5.1 depicts the temporal variation of annual case load, postoperative mortality, morbidity, and length of hospital stay in our series.

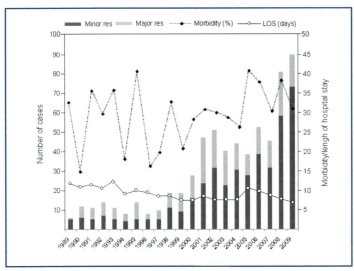

Fig. 5.1 Temporal variation of annual case load, postoperative morbidity, and length of hospital stay (*LOS*) in our series of patients undergoing minor or major resection

5.3
Long-term Results

5.3.1
Survival

Since 1990, single-institution series exceeding 100 patients have reported 5-year survival figures ranging from 25% to 58%. Despite the lack of level 1 evidence, the survival benefit of liver resection is no longer debated. A large series reported by Scheele et al. [24] clearly demonstrated improved survival following hepatectomy compared to patients with unresectable disease and to patients with resectable disease who did not undergo operation. In the group treated by potentially curative resection, 5- and 10-year survival rates of 40% and 27% were achieved. In contrast, median survivals of 6.9 months and 14.2 months were observed in the unresectable group and in the non-operative group with resectable disease, respectively, with no 5-year survivors. Table 5.2 reports the long-term results from major published series of hepatic resection for colorectal liver metastases [2-6, 14, 16-20] Despite expanding indications for resection to include patients with disease once deemed unresectable, 5-year overall survival is now consistently as high as 58%, as reported in single- and multi-institutional studies. In patients with solitary liver metastases, high survival rates of > 70% can be obtained [37]. These high survival rates reflect improvement in patient selection, perioperative and postoperative care, multidisciplinary treatment, and an appropriately aggressive approach to safe hepatic resection.

Table 5.2 Overall (OS) and disease free survival (DFS) after resection for colorectal liver metastases

Author	Year	Patients (n)	OS (years)				DFS		
			Median (months)	3 (%)	5 (%)	10 (%)	Median (months)	3-years (%)	5-years (%)
Scheele [2]	1995	496	-	-	39	24	-	-	34
Nordliger [3]	1996	1568	-	44	28	-	-	35	23
Fong [4]	1999	1001	42	57	37	22	-	-	-
Minagawa[5]	2000	235	-	51	38	26	15	30	26
Choti [6]	2002	226	46	57	40	26	16	63	28
Ercolani [7]	2002	245	-	53	34	-	-	-	-
Abdalla [17]	2004	190	-	73	58	-	-	40	32
Adam [8]	2004	335	-	66	48	30	-	30	22
Fernandez [9]	2004	100	-	66	59	-	-	35	35
Pawlik [18]	2005	557	74.3	74	58	-	-	-	-
Jonas [10]	2007	660	-	-	37	23	-	-	29
Malik [11]	2007	700	49.9	62	45	-	21	39	31
Tomlinson [12]	2007	612	44	-	-	16.6	-	-	-
Rees [14]	2008	929	42.5	-	36	23	23.4	-	24
Viganò [19]	2008	125	-	42	23	16	-	28.7	17
de Jong [20]	2009	1669	36	-	47.3	-	23	37.7	30
House [16]	2010	1600	53.5	63	44	-	22.5	36.5	30
Capussotti (*unpublished*)	2010	544[a]	-	89	47	-	-	62	37

[a]Data on patients who underwent resection after 1998

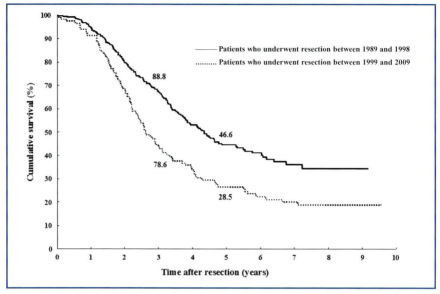

Fig. 5.2 Overall survival in our series of patients who underwent resection before ($n = 124$) and after ($n = 489$) 1999. A significant improvement in survival was observed despite more aggressive surgery

Consistent with previous findings [6, 16], in our series we observed a significantly improved patient survival in the most recent period (1999–2009). The 3- and 5-year survival estimates were 88.8% and 46.6% vs. 78.6% and 28.5% in the 124 patients who underwent resection before 1999 (Fig. 5.2).

5.3.2
Recurrence

Although advances in surgical and medical oncology have resulted in the prolongation of survival for patients with colorectal liver metastases, many patients still develop recurrent disease. Using a large multi-institutional database of 1669 patients treated with surgery (resection: 90.2%, resection plus radiofrequency ablation (RFA): 8.0%, or RFA alone: 1.8%), we recently analyzed the rates and patterns of recurrence [20]. While 5-year overall survival was 47.3%, more than 56% of patients suffered a recurrence, with a median recurrence-free survival (RFS) time of 16.3 months. The first site of recurrence was intrahepatic only (43.2% of patients), extrahepatic only (35.8%), or intra- and extrahepatic (21.0%). No difference was found in RFS based on the site of recurrence (intrahepatic: 16.9 months; extrahepatic 16.6 months; intra- and extrahepatic: 16.2 months). Interestingly, our result pointed out the importance of an integrated treatment since patients receiving adjuvant chemotherapy had a reduced overall recurrence risk. Conversely, RFA use and R1 margin status were predictive of intrahepatic recurrence. Therefore, whenever possible, a complete resection of all metastatic sites rather than a combination of treatments should be the surgical goal. Moreover, we were able to analyze the pattern of recurrence in a subgroup of 197 patients who underwent repeat curative intent surgery. This remained similar with regard to intrahepatic vs. extrahepatic vs. intrahepatic plus extrahepatic disease. In addition, the median RFS following repeat surgery was comparable to that after the first hepatectomy.

5.4
Prognostic Factors

Since the early 1980s, almost all studies reporting long-term survival after hepatic resection have attempted to identify potential determinants of outcome. Primary tumor features, characteristics of the liver metastases, presence or absence of extrahepatic disease, and the radicality of hepatic resection represent the factors most commonly found to be prognostic for clinical outcome (Table 5.3) [2-6, 11, 14, 19, 25-36]. However, a precise definition of the real survival impact of each of these factors is impossible. In fact, comparison between studies is generally limited, owing to differences in the categorization of single variables. For example, a definition of "synchronous metastases" is not given in most series, but could be 1, 3, or 6 months within resection of the primary tumor. Time interval between resection of the primary tumor and the metastases has also been classified using different cut-offs (4, 12, 24, and 30 months). Similarly, categories for number and size of liver metastases vary extremely, and reporting of the type of liver resection is inconsistent. In addition, results from multivariate analysis cannot be directly compared, as factors included in each model differ between studies.

One of the most relevant developments has been the recent shift from using prognostic factors to select patients for liver resection to using them to select patients for multimodality treatment. Today, negative prognostic factors are no longer used to deny patients a potentially curative resection, since the only contraindication to liver surgery is the impossibility to achieve a complete resection while preserving a sufficient liver remnant with adequate vascular inflow, outflow, and biliary drainage.

The following sections present an overview of the potential prognostic factors.

5.4.1
Traditional Prognostic Factors

Traditional prognosticators of poor outcome relate to the characteristics and extent of the disease and to perioperative factors. Notably, most of these were determined before the advent of effective systemic chemotherapy, and their utility as prognostic indicators in the era of modern chemotherapy is therefore unknown. Table 5.3 reports the significance of the most frequently identified prognostic factors in selected,

Table 5.3 Significance of prognostic factors for patient survival

Author	Year	Age	Sex	Site of primary tumor	Stage of primary tumor	CEA	Tumor size	Number of metastases	Synchronous	Bilobar distribution	Disease free interval	Extrahepatic disease	Type of resection	Narrow margin	Positive margin	Morbidity	R0	Adjuvant chemotherapy	Positive lymph nodes
Fortner [25]	1984	-	-	-	»	-	-	-			-								
Scheele [2]	1995	-	-	-	↑	-	↑	-	↑	-			+	-					
Nordlinger [3]	1996	-	-	+	↑	-	↑	↑	↑	-	↑	+	-	↑		↑	-		
Ohlsonn [26]	1998				-	↑	-	-				↑							+
Cady [27]	1998				-	↑	-	↑	-	-	-			+					
Fong [4]	1999	-	-	-	↑	↑	↑	+	-	+	↑	↑	+	↑			↑		
Ambiru [28]	1999	-	-	-	↑	-	-	↑	+	-			-	↑				↑	+
Iwatsuki [29]	1999	-	-	+			↑	↑		↑	↑	+	+	+	+		↑	-	+
Minagawa [5]	2000	-	-	-	↑	-	-	↑	-	-	-	-	-	-					↑
Ueno [30]	2000	-	-	-	↑	+	-	↑	-			↑	-						-
Lise [31]	2001	-	-	-	↑	-	↑	↑	-				-	↑		+	↑	-	
Choti [6]	2002				-	↑	-	-	-		-		-		↑				
Nagashima [32]	2004	-	-	-	-	-	↑	↑	-	-	-	↑							

Schindl [33]	2005	-	-	+	↑	↑	+	↑	-	-								↑	
Wei [34]	2006	+	-	-	↑		↑	↑	-	-					+				
Zakaria [35]	2007	-	-	+	↑	-	↑	-		-	↑			-			-		↑
Malik [11]	2007	-	-		-	-	+	↑	-		-					+		-	-
Rees [14]	2008	-	-	-	↑	↑	+	-	-	-	-	↑	-		↑		+	-	-
Vigano [19]	2008	-	↑	-	-		-	↑	↑	-	+	↑	-		↑	+			
Kishi [36]	2009	-	-		-	-	-	-			-		-		↑				
Rate of positivity (%)		6	6	20	65	41	55	60	23	13	40	70	25	75	85	100	100	14	63

The results of univariate (-, not significant; +, significant) and multivariate (↑, significant) analyses are reported. Empty space: factor not studied recent series involving more than 100 resected patients. The most striking finding is the inconsistency with which most of these factors are reported to adversely affect outcome. Table 5.3 shows for each factor the percentage of positivity, indicating the proportion of studies in which each characteristic was reported to be significant. In the following, we present available data relevant to a reframing of the discussion of prognostic factors vs. selection factors to define resectability.

Historically, patients who underwent resection of metastases with diameters > 4 or 5 cm were reported to have poorer survival rates. Recently, Minagawa et al. [5] showed that in 235 patients undergoing resection of colorectal liver metastases, maximum tumor diameter did not affect patient survival. Similarly, Hamady's group found that patients who underwent resection of metastases ≥ 8 cm had survival rates comparable to those of patients with smaller metastases [38]. Because of these conflicting results, tumor size cannot be accepted as a criterion for determining which patients should be operated. Size may negatively impact the surgeon's ability to gain negative margins or to leave an adequate remnant, but if a patient's disease is potentially resectable he or she should not be denied the opportunity to undergo complete resection. In addition, tumor size may be a function of when the tumor is found during the disease course, rather than a true predictor of biological aggressiveness.

Multiple metastases and the presence of bilobar disease are correlated with a less favorable prognosis compared to patients with a single metastatic site, since these features are associated with a higher risk of extrahepatic disease and a greater risk of systemic recurrence after surgery. However, controversies still exist as to whether the number of multiple tumors truly represents a significant prognostic factor. Kokudo et al. [39] found that the survival of patients with four or more metastases was similar to that of patients with fewer metastases. In addition, the maximum number of hepatic tumors in long-term survivors reported in the literature is constantly increasing, suggesting that a subset of patients with multiple nodules can be cured, especially when treated with a multimodality approach. Pawlik et al. [40], in a paper reporting on a cohort of 159 patients with more than four metastases treated with preoperative chemotherapy, found 5-year disease-free and overall survival rates of 22% and 51%, respectively, after hepatic resection. Similarly, Tanaka et al. [41] demonstrated that 5-year survival after resection was significantly better for those patients with multiple (5 or more) metastases treated with preoperative chemotherapy than for those who did not receive any preoperative treatment (38.9% vs. 20.7%). The definitive survival benefit of resection in patients with more than four metastases was recently demonstrated in a meta-analysis of all published series [42]. Therefore, the number of metastases should no longer be considered a contraindication for curative hepatic resection but rather a prognostic factor, which might be overcome by surgery and systemic chemotherapy. The limit on the number of resectable metastases has not yet been determined.

A short disease-free interval after resection of the primary tumor has been repeatedly reported to significantly impact survival [4, 29]. However, after controlling for competing factors other authors did not find a survival correlation [5]. Again, despite the potential for a much more guarded prognosis, early tumor relapse after the primary treatment should not contraindicate *de principe* liver resection.

Tumor marker assessment, specifically CEA, is routinely performed in the preoperative setting. However, the value of the serum CEA level with respect to prognosis remains unclear. While some authors did observe a significant correlation with poor outcome [4], many reports failed to demonstrate a clear survival disadvantage in patients with high plasma CEA concentrations prior to surgery [5].

The radicality of resection is probably the most important determinant of outcome. In a recent review of all published studies on surgical resection of colorectal liver metastases, the survival of patients undergoing R0 resections was substantially better (32% at 5 years) than that of patients undergoing R1 resections (7.2% at 5 years) [1]. In all published series, the commonest cause of R1 resection was tumor involvement of the surgical margins, as defined by the presence of tumor cells at the line of transection detected by histologic examination. While the importance of a radical (R0) resection is no longer disputed, much debate still exists regarding the significance of the negative margin width. A detailed examination of this issue is reported in Chapter 3 of this book.

Another, surgically related independent determinant of poor outcome is the amount of intraoperative blood loss; however, its importance is still controversial [43, 44]. Nonetheless, blood transfusions, which are strongly dependent on the amount of blood loss, have been shown to be a significant risk factor for poor outcome. In a series of 1351 patients who underwent resection for colorectal liver metastases, Kooby et al. [45] observed the greatest detrimental effect of blood transfusion during the perioperative course, where it was an independent predictor of operative mortality, complications, and length of hospital stay. This effect was dose-related. Patients receiving one or two units or more than two units of blood had an operative mortality of 2.5% and 11.1%, respectively, compared to 1.2% for patients not requiring transfusions. Transfusion was also associated with adverse long-term survival by univariate analysis, but this factor was not significant on multivariate analysis. Therefore, hemorrhage control, either with the use of different clamping methods, maintenance of a low central venous pressure, or a precise technique of parenchymal transection, is pivotal to optimize surgical outcome.

The prognostic significance of the presence of an extrahepatic disease and its clinical implications in terms of surgical indication and long-term outcome are extensively presented in Chapter 9 of this book.

Besides the above-mentioned factors, another interesting, independent prognostic indicator emerged in our recent analysis of a series of 121 patients with a complete 10-year follow-up [19]. Multivariate analysis revealed that postoperative morbidity was a significant risk factor for worse survival (HR 2.3). Similar results were obtained by Farid et al. [46] in a series of 705 consecutive patients undergoing resection for colorectal liver metastases. In their study, the 5-year disease-free and overall survival rates for those patients with ($n = 197$) or without ($n = 508$) complications were 13% vs. 26%, and 24% vs. 37%, respectively (all $p < 0.001$). In addition, multivariate analysis showed postoperative sepsis to be an independent factor associated with both disease-free and overall survival. Interestingly, the authors demonstrated that intra-abdominal and respiratory infections but not wound infections were associated with poorer long-term outcomes. The influence of morbidity on survival was reported for patients with esophageal, colorectal, and lung cancers. Surgical complications, specifically sepsis and liver insufficiency, prolong postoperative immunodepression and may lead to the proliferation of metastatic cells. In addition, liver insufficiency, usually caused by a small residual parenchyma, is associated with a greater regenerative stimulus that is sustained by an increased production of growth factors, a situation that might also favor neoplastic cell proliferation.

5.4.2
Scoring Systems

The expansion of indications for surgical resection in patients with colorectal liver metastases has increased the clinical heterogeneity among these individuals. Even though these patients are still uniformly grouped within AJCC/UICC stage IV, they may have variable disease characteristics that potentially influence their prognosis. Indeed, data from several studies indicate a multifactorial determinant of long-term outcome (Table 5.3). In an attempt to derive more prognostic information, some investigators have combined multiple clinicopathologic factors to formulate prognostic scoring systems. Predictive scoring models calculated on quantitative data have numerous benefits. Within these scoring systems, various patient- and tumor-related variables are considered in order to stratify patients according to their risk for disease recurrence and tumor-related death. Moreover, the stratification of patients into risk categories is helpful for comparison of patient cohorts among different studies and institutions.

Prognostic scoring for patients with colorectal liver metastases was first introduced in 1996 by Nordlinger et al. [3]. Using a large multicenter series of 1568 resected patients, the authors developed a system based on seven variables found to have an independent prognostic value: age > 60 years, primary tumor extension into the serosa, lymphatic spread of the primary tumor, time interval from primary tumor to metastases < 2 years, four or more metastases, size of the largest lesion ≥ 5 cm, and surgical margin < 1 cm. Since the relative risks associated with each of these factors were comparable, the authors assigned one point to each factor, to stratify the population into three risk groups: low risk (0–2 points), with an expected 2-year survival rate of 79%; intermediate risk (3–4 points), with an expected 2-year survival rate of 60%; and high risk (5–7 points), with an estimated 2-year survival rate of 43%.

Subsequently, two scoring systems were proposed in rapid succession. Iwatsuki et al. [29], in a single-institution study of 230 patients, devised a risk- score based on more than three hepatic metastases, size of metastasis > 8 cm, hepatic metastases confirmed within ≤ 30 months of the primary cancer, and bilobar hepatic metastases. Five risk grades were stratified based on the sum of the individual prognostic variables: grade 1 being no risk factor present to grade 5, which includes patients with four risk factors. However, it is the Clinical Risk Score of Fong et al. [4] that has rapidly gained wide acceptance. Using the same methodology as Nordlinger et al. [3], the authors analyzed 1001 consecutive patients operated for colorectal liver metastases at a single institution. The Clinical Risk Score (Table 5.4) is based on two imaging

5 Results of Surgery and Prognostic Factors

Table 5.4 The Clinical Risk Score (CRS). Survival stratified per CRS classes as reported by Fong et al. [4]. The CRS is calculated by summing the points (0 or 1) assigned to each clinical criterion

Clinical criteria	Point assigned		Score	Overall survival (years)		
	No	Yes		3 (%)	5 (%)	Median (months)
Node-positive primary	0	1	0	72	60	74
Disease-free interval < 12 months	0	1	1	66	44	51
Tumor number > 1	0	1	2	60	40	47
Tumor size > 5 cm	0	1	3	42	20	33
CEA > 200 ng/ml	0	1	4	38	25	20
			5	27	14	22

factors (number of metastases: single vs. multiple, and their size: ≤ 5 cm vs. >5 cm) and three oncological parameters (disease-free interval from the primary to discovery of the liver metastases >12 months vs. <12 months; CEA < 200 ng/ml vs. > 200 ng/ml; and node-positive primary tumor). The authors assigned to each criterion one point, and the total score was compared with the clinical outcome of each patient after liver resection. The total score was found to be highly predictive of long-term outcome, with median survival estimates of 74, 51, 47, 33, 20, and 22 months for patients with 0, 1, 2, 3, 4, and 5 points, respectively. Corresponding 5-year survival estimates decreased from 60% in the best prognostic group to 14% in those within the worst category.

More recently, the HPB Unit of Basingstoke, UK, proposed a similar, albeit more complex, prognostic score, the Basingstoke Predictive Index, in which each of its seven factors are appropriately weighted to provide an accurate prediction of cancer-specific survival [14]. As with other scoring systems from small study populations, its use remains so far anecdotal.

Despite the predictive value of each score within the original patient cohort, external validation of these scoring systems is still limited. In an ad hoc analysis, Zakaria et al. [35] investigated the prognostic stratification ability of the Nordlinger score, the Clinical Risk Score, and the Iwatsuki score in a series of 662 patients undergoing liver resection for colorectal metastases. Surprisingly, the authors reported no valid risk stratification of their patients with any of the assessed scores. However, since patients included in the analysis were operated on during the period 1960–1995, their treatment might not have reflected current standards of care. By contrast, using a cohort of 281 patients who underwent resection after 2002, Reissfelder et al.[47] demonstrated that two score systems, the Clinical Risk Score and the Iwatsuki score, significantly predicted the survival of patients undergoing current standards of therapy. However, the Clinical Risk Score did not show monotonicity of gradients, with patients in higher risk categories exhibiting improved survival compared to patients in lower risk categories. Therefore, its clinical utility remains controversial.

To further improve upon previous prognostic scoring systems, Kattan et al. [48] constructed a nomogram for predicting diseases-specific survival in the individual patient. Rather than count risk factors, a nomogram considers the specific value of each factor. Therefore, while it predicts survival more accurately, it is more specific to the individual patient. This nomogram can be downloaded into a PDA for routine use in the clinics or at the patient's bedside at www.nomograms.org .

5.4.3
Other Prognostic Factors

From the above discussion it appears that conventional clinicopathologic factors are somehow inadequate as prognostic indicators. Thus, there has been increased interest in identifying other prognostic factors, both clinical and, more recently, molecular, that may help in better defining patients at risk for disease recurrence after hepatic resection. These additional factors seem to more clearly define tumor biology.

5.4.3.1
Clinical and Pathologic Prognostic Factors

Response to chemotherapy, in terms of either tumor reduction/stabilization or tumor progression, is emerging as one of the most powerful prognostic factors. An aggressive tumor, suggested by the impossibility of its control with modern cytotoxic agents, has been advocated as a formal contraindication to liver resection [49]. However, several studies have shown that response to chemotherapy closely correlates with long term-survival and with a reduced risk of tumor recurrence after hepatic resection. In a recent study, Gruenberger et al. [50] found that a response to six cycles of XELOX or FOLFOX significantly improved an unfavorable prognosis, defined on the basis of established parameters (Clinical Risk Score) in more than two-thirds of the patients. Therefore, tumor response, traditionally evaluated by the magnitude of tumor volume reduction, may be considered an ideal parameter to estimate prognosis in patients diagnosed with metastatic colorectal cancer. However, size-based radiologic criteria, i.e., the Response Evaluation Criteria in Solid Tumors (RECIST), can be inadequate in defining tumor response, especially when biologics, which have a cytostatic mechanism of action, are used. In support of this, a recent phase 3 trial showed that the addition of bevacizumab to FOLFOX or XELOX improved progression-free survival (PFS) without affecting RECIST-defined response rates [51]. After bevacizumab-containing therapy, colorectal liver metastases tend to decrease in size and to undergo unique morphologic changes, as observed by computed tomography, which shows a transformation to homogeneous, hypoattenuating lesions with well-defined borders without a rim of enhancement.

Response defined on the basis of these characteristics has been shown to significantly correlate with both the percentage of residual tumor cells and survival. By contrast, RECIST criteria were less closely correlated with pathologic response and did not predict survival in resected or unresected disease [52].

Similar to the clinical response, the pathologic response to chemotherapy has been recently recognized as one of the most important prognostic factors. This is consistent with findings observed in patients treated with preoperative chemotherapy for other cancer types such as breast, esophageal, gastric, and colorectal cancers. In a recent European study, Rubbia-Brandt et al. [53] reported a significant correlation between histologic response to chemotherapy and overall survival in 112 patients primarily treated with oxaliplatin-based chemotherapy. Using Tumor Regression Grading (TRG), which is a modification of Mandard's scheme for the assessment of pathologic response to neoadjuvant treatments in esophageal carcinomas, the authors demonstrated that, compared with tumors not treated with preoperative chemotherapy, tumors treated with preoperative chemotherapy exhibit significant regression, with marked reduction or disappearance of viable tumor cells and fibrosis overgrowth but not an increase of necrosis. Oxaliplatin appeared to add substantial efficacy to FU and irinotecan regimens in terms of histologic tumor regression and clinical outcome. Subsequently, Blazer III et al. [54] evaluated the long-term prognostic significance of pathologic response in a larger series of 305 patients who had undergone resection and were treated with preoperative irinotecan- or oxaliplatin-based chemotherapy. Using a different method to assess tumor response, defined semi-quantitatively as the percentage of residual tumor cells relative to the total tumor surface area, they showed a major response (i.e. < 50% viable tumor cells) in 36% of the specimen as well as a 5-year survival of 41% for patients treated with irinotecan-based regimens and 43% for patients treated with oxaliplatin-based chemotherapy, without significant survival difference between regimens. Significant predictors of a major response were preoperative CEA level < 5 ng/mL, tumor size < 3 cm, and chemotherapy combining oxaliplatin and bevacizumab. Therefore due to its prognostic relevance, pathologic response should now be routinely included in the pathology report.

The histopathologic characteristics of treated and untreated metastases might influence their ultrasound echogenicity. De Oliveira et al. [55], in a prospective study of 84 hepatic resections for colorectal metastases, showed that patients with a hypoechoic lesion, as shown by intraoperative ultrasonography, had a significantly shorter median survival (30.2 months) than patients who had either isoechoic (53.2 months) or hyperechoic (42.3 months) lesions. Consistently, 5-year survival was also associated with the echogenic appearance of the lesions (hypoechoic 14.4% vs. isoechoic 37.4% vs. hyperechoic 46.2%). Although the authors did not compare the intraoperative findings with tumor histology, they speculated that intratumoral biologic characteristics, such as mucin, or fibrosis, contribute to a lesion's echogenicity which, in turn, is associated with its prognosis. Yet, further studies are needed.

Another new and interesting prognostic indicator is the host's inflammatory response to tumor (IRT) [11]. Recent studies have shown that, in a number of malignancies including colorectal carcinoma, an IRT before surgery correlates with a poor cancer-specific survival. The presence of an IRT, defined by an elevated preoperative C-reactive protein (CRP) (> 10 mg/L) or a neutrophil to lymphocyte ratio (NLR) > 5, may simply reflect nonspecific inflammation secondary to tumor necrosis or local tissue damage. But, it may also reflect a favorable environment for the establishment and growth of metastases. In fact, the serum level of angiogenic vascular endothelial growth factor is increased in the presence of elevated CRP. In addition, an inverse relationship has been shown between the level of CRP and the infiltration of lymphocytes at the periphery of the tumor [56]. A weak lymphocytic infiltration at the tumor margin, reflecting an impaired host immune response, has been shown to predict poor prognosis in patients who had resection for colorectal liver metastases [57]. The inflammatory response suggested by the CRP level or the NLR is a useful indicator because it can be easily measured with a preoperative blood sampling. The prognostic significance of the NLR and of its changes after chemotherapy was recently confirmed by Kishi et al. [36]. In their study, the authors showed that NLR > 5 independently predicted worse survival in patients treated with chemotherapy followed or not by hepatic resection. Interestingly, when chemotherapy normalized high NLR, improved survival was observed. In addition, NLR at multivariate analysis overshadowed all other established prognostic factors, such as those included in the Clinical Risk Score (lymph node metastasis, disease-free interval < 1 year, CEA > 200 ng/ml, tumor size > 5 cm, and multiple tumors). This result suggests that high NLR reflects an aggressive tumor biology associated with poor outcomes that cannot be estimated on the basis of previously proposed risk factors.

5.4.3.2
Molecular Markers

Specific molecular markers of various aspects of tumor biology have been shown to correlate with outcome. Proliferation markers, such as Ki-67 labeling index, tritiated thymidine uptake, and thymidylate synthase expression as well as microvessel density and thrombospondin-1, have been shown to be independent predictors of recurrence and survival [58]. Validation of other markers, notably p53 expression, has been limited by a failure of methodologies to account for their biological complexity. Among these various molecular markers, hTERT (human telomerase reverse transcriptase) expression has been extensively studied. Telomerase is expressed in most human tumors, resulting in stabilized telomere length and cell immortalization. Primary colon carcinoma hTERT status has been shown to correlate with overall survival. In a multi-institutional study, Domont et al. [59] demonstrated that positive hTERT nucleolar staining independently predicts overall survival in patients with surgically resected hepatic colorectal metastases, along with the number of metastases and the disease-free interval. Patients with none or one of these factors had a 5-year survival rate of 48%, whereas those with two or three factors had a 5-year survival of 15%.

New molecular techniques have demonstrated the presence of occult tumor cells in different body compartments (e.g., blood, bone marrow, or lymph nodes) after the resection of solid tumors [60]. The relationship between circulating tumor cells and the development of metastatic disease is still unclear. Tumor cell shedding into the peripheral circulation appears to be a relatively common event, but most of these cells do not survive [61]. However, in the appropriate environment, a large hematogenous bolus of viable tumor cells may give rise to distant metastases. Major hepatic resections are associated with profound immunologic changes and with the activation of clotting factors, which might enhance the metastatic potential of tumor cells disseminated during surgery. In a recent study, Kock et al. [62] showed that intraoperative tumor cell dissemination in blood and tumor cell detection in bone marrow are independent prognostic factors for disease-free survival in patients undergoing curative resection for colorectal liver metastases. Interestingly, all patients with detectable tumor cells in postoperative blood samples developed tumor recurrence. The authors also speculated that intraoperative tumor manipulation enhances the release of malignant cells, which in turn cause intrahepatic or extrahepatic tumor recurrence. The results of these studies need further confirmation but might prompt development of surgical strategies to prevent intraoperative hematogenous tumor cell shedding.

References

1. Simmonds PC, Primrose JN, Colquitt JL et al (2006) Surgical resection of hepatic metastases from colorectal cancer: A systematic review of published studies. Br J Cancer 94:982-999
2. Scheele J, Stang R, Altendorf-Hofmann A, Paul M (1995). Resection of colorectal liver metastases. World J Surg 19:59-71
3. Nordlinger B, Guiguet M, Vaillant JC et al (1996) Surgical resection of colorectal carcinoma metastases to the liver. A prognostic scoring system to improve case selection, based on 1568 patients. Association Francaise de Chirurgie. Cancer 77:1254-1262
4. Fong Y, Fortner J, Sun RL et al (1999) Clinical score for predicting recurrence after hepatic resection for metastatic colorectal cancer: analysis of 1001 consecutive cases. Ann Surg 230:309-318
5. Minagawa M, Makuuchi M, Torzilli G et al (2000) Extension of the frontiers of surgical indications in the treatment of liver metastases from colorectal cancer: long-term results. Ann Surg 231:487-99
6. Choti MA, Sitzmann JV, Tiburi MF et al (2002) Trends in long-term survival following liver resection for hepatic colorectal metastases. Ann Surg 235:759-766
7. Ercolani G, Grazi GL, Ravaioli M et al (2002) Liver resection for multiple colorectal metastases. Influence of parenchymal involvement and total tumor volume, vs number or location, on long-term survival. Arch Surg 137:1187-1192
8. Adam R, Delvart V, Pascal G et al (2004) Rescue surgery for unresectable colorectal liver metastases downstaged by chemotherapy. A model to predict long-term survival. Ann Surg 240: 644–658
9. Fernandez FG, Drebin JA, Linehan DC et al (2004) Five-year survival after resection of hepatic metastases from colorectal cancer in patients screened by positron emission tomography with F-18 fluorodeoxyglucose (FDG-PET). Ann Surg 240:438-447
10. Jonas S, Thelen A, Benckert C et al (2007) Extended resections of liver metastases from colorectal cancer. World J Surg 31:511–521

11. Malik HZ, Prasad R, Halazun KJ et al (2007) Preoperative prognostic score for predicting survival after hepatic resection for colorectal liver metastases. Ann Surg 246:806–814
12. Tomlinson JS, Jarnagin WR, DeMatteo RP et al (2007) Actual 10-year survival after resection of colorectal liver metastases defines cure. J Clin Oncol 25:4575-4580
13. Are C, Gonen M, Zazzali K et al (2007) The impact of margins on outcome after hepatic resection for colorectal metastasis. Ann Surg 246:295–300
14. Rees M, Tekkis PP, Welsh FKS et al (2008) Evaluation of long-term survival after hepatic resection for metastatic colorectal cancer. A multifactorial model of 929 patients. Ann Surg 247: 125–135
15. Gold JS, Are C, Kornprat P et al (2008) Liver metastases from colorectal cancer is associated with improved mortality without change in oncologic outcome. Trends in treatment over time in 440 patients. Ann Surg 247: 109–117
16. House MG, Ito H, Gönen M et al (2010) Survival after hepatic resection for metastatic colorectal cancer: trends in outcomes for 1,600 patients during two decades at a single institution. J Am Coll Surg 210:744-754
17. Abdalla EK, Vauthey JN, Ellis LM et al (2004) Recurrence and outcomes following hepatic resection, radiofrequency ablation, and combined resection/ablation for colorectal liver metastases. Ann Surg 239:818-825
18. Pawlik TM, Scoggins CR, Zorzi D et al (2005) Effect of surgical margin status on survival and site of recurrence after hepatic resection for colorectal metastases. Ann Surg 241:715-724
19. Viganò L, Ferrero A, Lo Tesoriere R et al (2008) Liver surgery for colorectal metastases: results after 10 years of follow-up. Long-term survivors, late recurrences, and prognostic role of morbidity. Ann Surg Oncol 15:2458-2464
20. de Jong MC, Pulitano C, Ribero D et al (2009) Rates and patterns of recurrence following curative intent surgery for colorectal liver metastasis. An international multi-institutional analysis of 1669 patients. Ann Surg 250:440–448
21. Mullen JT, Ribero D, Reddy S et al (2007) Hepatic insufficiency and mortality in 1059 non-cirrhotic patients undergoing major hepatectomy. J Am Coll Surg 204:854–864
22. Capussotti L, Viganò L, Giuliante F et al (2009) Liver dysfunction and sepsis determine operative mortality after liver resection. Br J Surg 96:88-94
23. Jarnagin WR, Gonen M, Fong Y et al (2002) Improvement in perioperative outcome after hepatic resection. Analysis of 1,803 consecutive cases over the past decade. Ann Surg 236:397–407
24. Scheele J, Altendorf-Hofmann A (1999) Resection of colorectal liver metastases. Langenbeck's Arch Surg 384:313–327
25. Fortner JG, Silva JS, Golbey RB et al (1984) Multivariate analysis of a personal series of 247 consecutive patients with liver metastases from colorectal cancer. I. Treatment by hepatic resection. Ann Surg 199:306-316
26. Ohlsson B, Stenram U, Tranberg KG (1998) Resection of colorectal metastases: 25-year experience. World J Surg 22:268 –276
27. Cady B, Jenkins RL, Steele GD Jr et al (1998) Surgical margin in hepatic resection for colorectal metastasis: a critical and improvable determinant of outcome. Ann Surg 227:566 –571
28. Ambiru S, Miyazaki M, Isono T et al (1999) Hepatic resection for colorectal metastases. Analysis of prognostic factors. Dis Colon Rectum 42:632-639
29. Iwatsuki S, Dvorchik I, Madariaga JR et al (1999) Hepatic resection for metastatic colorectal adenocarcinoma: a proposal of a prognostic scoring system. J Am Coll Surg 189:291-299
30. Ueno H, Mochizuki H, Hatsuse K et al (2000) Indicators for treatment strategies of colorectal liver metastases. Ann Surg 231:59–66
31. Lise M, Bacchetti S, Da Pian P et al (2001) Patterns of recurrence after resection of colorectal liver metastases: prediction by models of outcome analysis. World J Surg 25:638–644
32. Nagashima I, Takada T, Matsuda K et al (2004) A new scoring system to classify patients with colorectal liver metastases: proposal of criteria to select candidates for hepatic resection. J Hepatobiliary Pancreat Surg 11:79–83

5 Results of Surgery and Prognostic Factors

33. Schindl M, Wigmore SJ, Currie EJ et al (2005) Prognostic scoring in colorectal cancer liver metastases. Development and validation. Arch Surg 140:183-189
34. Wei AC, Greig PD, Grant D et al (2006) Survival after hepatic resection for colorectal metastases: a 10-year experience. Ann Surg Oncol 13:668-676
35. Zakaria S, Donohue JH, Que FG, et al (2007) Hepatic resection for colorectal metastases: value for risk scoring systems? Ann Surg 246:183-191
36. Kishi Y, Kopetz S, Chun YS et al (2009) Blood neutrophil-to-lymphocyte ratio predicts survival in patients with colorectal liver metastases treated with systemic chemotherapy. Ann Surg Oncol 16:614–622
37. Aloia TA, Vauthey JN, Loyer EM et al (2007) Solitary colorectal liver metastasis. Resection determines outcome. Arch Surg 141:460-467
38. Hamady ZZ, Malik HZ, Finch R et al (2006) Hepatic resection for colorectal metastasis: impact of tumour size. Ann Surg Oncol 13:1493-1439
39. Kokudo N, Imamura H, Sugawara Y et al (2004) Surgery for multiple hepatic colorectal metastases. J Hepatobiliary Pancreat Surg 11:84-91
40. Pawlik TM, Abdalla EK, Ellis LM et al (2006) Debunking dogma: surgery for four or more colorectal liver metastases is justified. J Gastrointest Surg 10:240-248
41. Tanaka K, Adam R, Shimada H et al (2003) Role of neoadjuvant chemotherapy in the treatment of multiple colorectal metastases to the liver. Br J Surg 90: 963–969
42. Smith MD McCall JL (2009) Systematic review of tumour number and outcome after radical treatment of colorectal liver metastases. Br J Surg 96:1101-1113
43. Kooby DA, Stockman J, Ben-Porat L et al (2003) Influence of transfusions on perioperative and long-term outcome in patients following hepatic resection for colorectal metastases. Ann Surg 237:860-869
44. Okano T, Ohwada S, Nakasone Y et al (2001) Blood transfusion causes deterioration in liver regeneration after partial hepatectomy in rats. J Surg Res 101:157-165
45. Kooby DA, Stockman J, Ben-Porat L et al (2003) Influence of transfusions on perioperative and long-term outcome in patients following hepatic resection for colorectal metastases. Ann Surg 237:860–870
46. Farid SG, Aldouri A, Morris-Stiff G et al (2010) Correlation between postoperative infective complications and long-term outcomes after hepatic resection for colorectal liver metastasis. Ann Surg 251:91–100
47. Reissfelder C, Rahbari NN, Koch M et al (2009) Validation of prognostic scoring systems for patients undergoing resection of colorectal cancer liver metastases. Ann Surg Oncol 16:3279–3288
48. Kattan MW, Gonen M, Jarnagin WR et al (2008) A nomogram for predicting disease-specific survival after hepatic resection for metastatic colorectal cancer. Ann Surg 247:282–287
49. Adam R, Pascal G, Castaing D et al (2004) Tumor progression while on chemotherapy. A contraindication to liver resection for multiple colorectal metastases? Ann Surg 240:1052–1064
50. Gruenberger B, Scheithauer W, Punzengruber R et al (2008) Importance of response to neoadjuvant chemotherapy in potentially curable colorectal cancer liver metastases. BMC Cancer 8:120
51. Saltz LB, Clarke S, Diaz-Rubio E et al (2008) Bevacizumab in combination with oxaliplatin-based chemotherapy as first-line therapy in metastatic colorectal cancer: a randomized phase III study. J Clin Oncol 26:2013-2019
52. Chun YS, Vauthey JN, Boonsirikamchai P et al. (2009) Association of computed tomography morphologic criteria with pathologic response and survival in patients treated with bevacizumab for colorectal liver metastases. JAMA 302:2338-2344
53. Rubbia-Brandt L, Giostra E, Brezault C et al (2007) Importance of histological tumor response assessment in predicting the outcome in patients with colorectal liver metastases treated with neo-adjuvant chemotherapy followed by liver surgery. Ann Oncol 18:299-304

54. Blazer DG III, Kishi Y, Maru DM et al (2008) Pathologic response to preoperative chemotherapy: a new outcome end point after resection of hepatic colorectal metastases. J Clin Oncol 26:5344-5351
55. DeOliveira ML, Pawlik TM, Gleisner AL et al (2007) Echogenic appearance of colorectal liver metastases on intraoperative ultrasonography is associated with survival after hepatic resection. J Gastrointest Surg 11:970-976
56. Canna K, McArdle PA, McMillan DC et al (2005) The relationship between tumor T-lymphocyte infiltration, the systemic inflammatory response and survival in patients undergoing curative resection for colorectal cancer. Br J Cancer 92:651-654
57. Okano K, Maeba T, Modoguchi A et al (2003) Lymphocytic infiltration surrounding liver metastases from colorectal cancer. J Surg Oncol 82:28-33
58. Neal CP, Garcea G, Doucas H et al (2006) Molecular prognostic markers in resectable colorectal liver metastases: a systematic review. Eur J Cancer 42:1728-1743
59. Domont J, Pawlik TM, Boige V et al (2005) Catalytic subunit of human telomerase reverse transcriptase is an independent predictor of survival in patients undergoing curative resection of hepatic colorectal metastases: a multicenter analysis. J Clin Oncol 23:3086-3093
60. Pantel K, von Knebel Doeberitz M (2000) Detection and clinical relevance of micrometastatic cancer cells. Curr Opin Oncol 12:95–101
61. Liotta LA, Stetler-Stevenson WG (1991) Tumor invasion and metastasis: an imbalance of positive and negative regulation. Cancer Res 51(suppl 18): 5054–5059
62. Koch M, Kienle P, Hinz U et al (2005) Detection of hematogenous tumor cell dissemination predicts tumor relapse in patients undergoing surgical resection of colorectal liver metastases. Ann Surg 241:199–205

Preoperative Chemotherapy

6

Abstract Oxaliplatin and irinotecan have widened the chemotherapy alternatives available to patients with metastatic colorectal cancer, and effective targeted agents have further improved treatment efficacy. Combinations of these drugs have set a new benchmark of survival at ~20 months, enabling a substantial number of patients who were not candidates for resection to qualify for the procedure. Liver resection after tumor downsizing has yielded encouraging results, although cure is rarely achieved. Based on several theoretical advantages, preoperative chemotherapy is increasingly being used also in patients with resectable disease. However, the debate is still ongoing especially with respect to the oncologic benefits and the numerous drawbacks, including hepatic toxicity and the risk of inducing a complete radiologic response.

6.1
Introduction

Since the life expectancy for individuals with untreated metastatic colorectal cancer is extremely poor, medical or surgical treatments are commonly offered to stage IV patients to prolong survival and enhance the quality of life. Although complete surgical resection is the only potentially curative treatment modality, at diagnosis 80% of patients are not considered to be candidates for resection because of the size, location, and extent of their disease. For these patients chemotherapy remains the only option. Over the past few years, exciting progress has occurred in the establishment of new standards in the treatment of patients with metastatic colorectal cancer. This chapter outlines the treatment options for patients with unresectable disease and addresses issues regarding preoperative chemotherapy in patients eligible for resection.

M. Aglietta (✉)
Medical Oncology, University of Turin, Division of Medical Oncology, Institute for Cancer Research and Treatment, Candiolo (TO), Italy

Surgical Treatment of Colorectal Liver Metastases. Lorenzo Capussotti (Ed.)
© Springer-Verlag Italia 2011

6.2
Unresectable Liver Metastases

The 21st century has heralded a new era in the treatment of metastatic colorectal cancer patients. From the late 1950s until recently, fluorouracil (FU) was the only available chemotherapeutic agent with demonstrated efficacy. However, response rates and median survival hovered at 10–15% and 10 months, respectively, affording treated patients minimal improvement in survival over supportive care. This response rate was improved to nearly 25% when leucovorin (LV) was used to modulate FU. Recently, four drugs have expanded, in relatively rapid succession, the armamentarium of agents active against colorectal cancer. When incorporated into FU/LV-based regimens, irinotecan and oxaliplatin have been shown to improve the response rate to approximately 50%. In addition, these combinations have set a new benchmark for survival at ~20 months [1-6]. The addition to standard combination therapy regimens of biological agents, such as monoclonal antibodies against vascular endothelial growth factor A (VEGF-A) and epidermal growth factor receptor (EGFR), has also been associated with increased response rates and improved survival. In the following, the use of these newer cytotoxic chemotherapies and biologic agents is discussed.

6.2.1
Conventional Chemotherapy

Several phase III trials have demonstrated that first-line multiagent chemotherapy, including irinotecan or oxaliplatin with infusional FU/LV consistently improves the response rate, time to progression, and median survival over FU/LV alone [1, 2, 5, 6]. Level I evidence also indicates that FOLFIRI (FU/LV plus irinotecan) and FOLFOX (FU/LV plus oxaliplatin) have equal activity and efficacy, with patient outcome not affected by the sequence of irinotecan and oxaliplatin administration [4]. In a combined analysis of seven recent randomized phase III trials, Grothey et al. [7] demonstrated that overall survival (OS) was tightly correlated with having received all three drugs in the course of the disease, independent of the order in which they were administered. In order to expose all patients to the three cytotoxics, the triplet regimen FOLFOXIRI (FU/LV, oxaliplatin, and irinotecan) has been used as a first-line treatment. In the GONO phase III trial, FOLFOXIRI, although moderately more toxic than FOLFIRI, proved to significantly increase progression-free survival (PFS) and OS [8]. Another relevant pharmacological advance is the availability of the oral fluoropyrimidine capecitabine. A meta-analysis of the studies comparing capecitabine plus oxaliplatin (CAPOX) with FOLFOX demonstrated that capecitabine is not inferior to FU in terms of PFS and OS [9]. Conversely, the results reported with capecitabine plus irinotecan (CAPIRI) are controversial.

With the increased number of first- and second-line treatment options, the major challenge has become how to best incorporate these drugs into treatment plans for individual patients. Treatment decision should consider the type of agent/s based on the efficacy and the toxicity profile, and the optimal scheme of administration (i.e., sequential therapy or combination therapy with doublets or triplets and continuous treatment until disease progression or intermittent administration, the so-called "stop-and-go" strategy). Yet, to define the optimal strategy, physicians must consider patient-specific factors. In patients with unresectable disease that will never become resectable (Fig. 6.1a), the aim of treatment is prolonging OS and achieving effective palliation of symptoms and a positive impact on the quality of life. An in-depth analysis of the factors guiding the therapeutic choice in such patients is beyond the scope of this chapter. Instead, we focus on patients with "potentially resectable" disease (Fig. 6.1b). This new category of patients has recently emerged as a consequence of the ability of newer chemotherapy regimens to downsize tumors and thus enable surgery that was not initially possible. In these patients, the objective of chemotherapy has therefore shifted from palliation to maximization of response rates. In fact, Folprecht et al. [10], based on data from retrospective studies and published trials, demonstrated a strong correlation between response rates and resection in patients with isolated liver metastases as well as in non-selected patients with metastatic disease. Data from several phase III trials have shown that response rates of approximately 50% can be obtained using doublets including irinotecan or oxali-

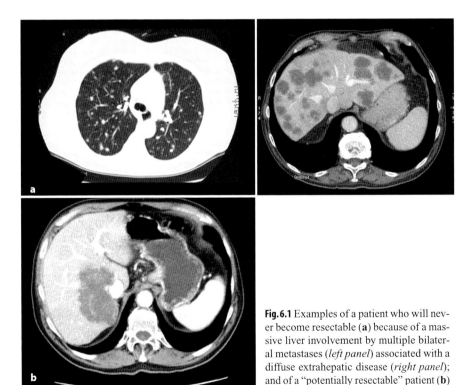

Fig. 6.1 Examples of a patient who will never become resectable (**a**) because of a massive liver involvement by multiple bilateral metastases (*left panel*) associated with a diffuse extrahepatic disease (*right panel*); and of a "potentially resectable" patient (**b**)

platin [1-6]. These two drugs were directly compared in a prospective randomized study allocating patients to FOLFIRI followed by FOLFOX6 or to the reverse sequence [4]. Objective response rates after first-line FOLFIRI and FOLFOX6 were similar (56% and 54%, respectively) with a non-significant advantage for FOLFOX as second-line therapy (15% vs. 4% for FOLFIRI). Using the triplets (FOLFOXIRI), Falcone et al. [8] showed a response rate of 60%. Due to the equivalence of irinotecan- and oxaliplatin-based regimens in terms of efficacy, treatment decision for first-line therapy, even in the neoadjuvant setting, can be made according to the toxicity profile of individual drugs or to personal preference. Moreover, since optimization of the preoperative regimen is critical to the success of downsizing unresectable metastases to a resectable situation, additional therapeutic strategies, such as use of targeted therapies and intra-arterial chemotherapy, may be utilized to further improve response rates.

6.2.2
The Role of Targeted Therapies

Basic science studies have identified molecular sites in tumor tissue that may serve as specific targets for treatment. The goal of this therapeutic strategy is the interruption of cellular pathways essential for tumor growth, survival, and metastasis. Currently, two classes of targeted compounds have been introduced into the clinical management of advanced colorectal cancer: EGFR antagonists and angiogenesis inhibitors.

Cetuximab, a chimeric monoclonal antibody against the extracellular binding domain of EGFR, is the first such inhibitor to be approved for the treatment of metastatic colorectal cancer. Initial studies with anti-EGFR antibodies were conducted in chemorefractory patients, in whom cetuximab was shown to improve response rates and PFS. These experiences were confirmed in the first-line setting. The CRYSTAL study [11] evaluated FOLFIRI plus cetuximab vs. FOLFIRI alone in 1217 patients. Response rates were significantly higher among patients receiving cetuximab (46.9% vs. 38.7%). In combination with FOLFOX, cetuximab was compared with FOLFOX alone in the randomized phase II OPUS study [12]: the addition of cetuximab to chemotherapy resulted in higher, albeit not significantly, activity (response rate 45.6% vs. 35.7%). In a recent study (the CELIM trial), Folprecht et al. [13] compared the efficacy of cetuximab in association with either FOLFOX6 or FOLFIRI and found that tumor response rate, which was the primary endpoint, was not statistically different in the two arms (68% and 57%, respectively). However, recent insight into EGFR biology has restricted the benefit of cetuximab to a specific subgroup of patients. In fact, the most relevant finding of translational research has been the identification of the mutational status of the *k-ras* gene, which encodes a G-protein involved in the downstream signaling of EGFR, as a predictor of resistance to anti-EGFR antibodies. Mutations in the *k-ras* gene occur in around 40% of colorectal tumors and result in a constitutively activated protein that is not affected by antibody binding at the extracellular EGFR domain. The single nucleotide point mutations in *k-ras* occur mostly in codons 12 (in 80% of the cases) and 13 of exon 2; less frequently (approximately 1% of all *k-ras* mutations), mutations involve codons 61, 146, or 154. The first report of a significant association between *k-ras* mutations and resistance to cetuximab has been subsequently confirmed by almost all retrospective investigations. In the CRYSTAL study, the subgroup of patients with wild-type *k-ras* who were treated with cetuximab had a significantly better response rate than the group receiving FOLFIRI alone (59.3% vs. 43.3%) [11]. Likewise, in the OPUS trial, the benefit of cetuximab was concentrated in the *k-ras* wild-type subgroup, with a response rate of 60.7% for cetuximab + FOLFOX4 compared to 37.0% for FOLFOX4 alone.

Bevacizumab is a humanized antibody targeting VEGF-A. It is an angiogenesis inhibitor that has been shown to improve OS when combined with chemotherapy in the first- or second-line treatment of patients with metastatic colorectal cancer. Clinical trials have shown that bevacizumab in combination with standard chemotherapy has an established, well tolerated, and consistent safety profile. Data from phase II and III trials indicated that the addition of bevacizumab to chemotherapy increases response rates by approximately 10% compared with chemotherapy alone, either with FU/LV (AVF2192g study) or with irinotecan-based (AVF2107 study) [14] or oxaliplatin-based doublets (NO16966 study) [15]. In a recent multicenter phase II study including exclusively patients with unresectable liver-only metastatic colorectal cancer, bevacizumab in combination with oxaliplatin and capecitabine, yielded a response rate of 78% and a 32% rate of conversion to resectable disease [16]. An identical response rate (77%) was obtained when bevacizumab was used in combination with FOLFOXIRI [17]. Moreover, bevacizumab is the only biological agent proven to confer an OS advantage to first-line chemotherapy with FU/LV and irinotecan in unselected patients [14]. Similarly, when added to XELOX or FOLFOX chemotherapy, bevacizumab has been shown to significantly prolong PFS.

In first-line treatment, most trials obtained higher response rates with cetuximab-based regimens than with bevacizumab-based regimens. As such, many clinicians prefer using cetuximab in patients with "potentially resectable" tumors expressing *k-ras* wild type. However, this choice is supported only by retrospective cross-study comparisons. Given the lack of cross-study standardization for the selection of patients for liver surgery after neoadjuvant chemotherapy, the definite benefit of cetuximab over bevacizumab in this subset of patients remains to be established. Ongoing studies, such as the Cancer and Leukemia Group B 80405 study, comparing chemotherapy plus either bevacizumab, cetuximab or both in *k-ras* wild type tumors, will provide useful data. In the meantime, further refinements in our capacity to predict resistance to cetuximab –evaluation of BRAF V600E mutation appears to be the most promising predictive factor– will help us to select patients who will likely benefit the most from cetuximab-containing regimens. A summary of response rates observed after preoperative chemotherapy with or without the addition of biologics is provided in Table 6.1.

Table 6.1 Preoperative chemotherapy with or without biologic agents, and secondary resection rates in patients with initially unresectable colorectal metastases

Author	Study	Type of study	N of patients (resected /initial)	Regimen	Response rate (%)	Resection rate (%)[a]	R0 resection rate (%)[a]
Giachetti et al [23]	—	Retrospective[b]	58/151	FU/LV + oxaliplatin (83% chronomodulated)	—	38	—
Rivoire et al [33]	—	Retrospective[b]	33/131	FU/LV or FOLFOX	—	25	—
Adam et al [24]	—	Retrospective	138/1104	FU/LV + oxaliplatin or irinotecan or both (87% chronomodulated)	—	12.5	11.7
Capussotti et al [35]	—	Retrospective	34/104	FOLFOX	—	32.7	26.9
Barone et al [25]	—	Phase II[b]	13/40	FU/LV + irinotecan	47.5	33	33
Alberts et al [26]	—	Phase II[b]	17/42	FOLFOX4	60	40	33.3
Saltz et al [1]	—	Phase III	na/226 na/226 na/231	Irinotecan alone FU/LV Irinotecan + bolus FU/LV	29 28 50	— — —	— — —
Perez-Staub et al [27]	OPTIMOX-1	Phase III	101/620	FOLFOX4 or «stop-and-go» FOLFOX7	—	16	—
Tournigand et al [4]	—	Phase III	10/109 24/111	FOLFIRI followed by FOLFOX FOLFOX followed by FOLFIRI	56 54	9 22	7 13
Falcone et al [8]	—	Phase III	18/122 7/122	FOLFOXIRI FOLFIRI	66 41	— —	15 (36)[c] 6 (12)[c]

Van Cutsem et al [11]	CRYSTAL	Phase III	42/599	FOLFIRI + cetuximab	46.9 (59.3)[d]	7	4.8
			22/599	FOLFIRI	38.7 (43.3)[d]	3.7	1.7
Bokemeyer et al [12]	OPUS	Phase II	na/170	FOLFOX + cetuximab	45.5 (60.7)[d]	6.5	4.7
			na/168	FOLFOX	35.7 (37)[d]	3.6	1.7
Folprecht et al [13]	CELIM Trial	Phase II [b]	20/56	FOLFOX6 + cetuximab	68	38	—
			16/55	FOLFIRI+ cetuximab	57	30	—
Hurwitz et al [14]	AVF2107	Phase III	na/402	Irinotecan + FU/LV + bevacizumab	44.8	—	—
			na/411	Irinotecan + FU/LV	34.8	—	—
Saltz et al [15]	NO16966	Phase III	59/699	FOLFOR or XELOX + bevacizumab	47	8,4	—
			43/701	FOLFOR or XELOX	49	6.1	—
Van Cutsem et al [28]	BEAT trial	Phase III	99/949	FOLFOX or XELOX + bevacizumab	—	10.4	8
			43/682	FOLFIRI + bevacizumab	—	6.5	5.1

na, Not available

[a] Percentage calculated on the entire series

[b] Studies or [c]subgroup analyses including only patients with liver-only metastases

[d] Data in *k-ras* wild-type patients

6.2.3
Intra-arterial Chemotherapy

The delivery of chemotherapy to the liver via the hepatic artery has the advantage of a higher chemotherapy exposure of the tumor over a longer period of time. Hepatic arterial infusion (HAI) chemotherapy, mainly using fluorodeoxyuridine (FUDR), has been a widely studied approach [18]. High response rates have been reported with 35 to 83% of patients having an objective radiologic response [19]. In patients with unresectable disease, this treatment has been compared in multiple studies to systemic therapy with FU or no therapy. In 1996, a meta-analysis of the published randomized trials demonstrated an improvement in response rate and a 27% relative survival advantage [20]. However, a subsequent randomized trial did not demonstrate improved survival compared to control arms [21]. In addition, HAI is limited by technical problems related to catheters, arterial ports, and implantable pumps. Newer forms of combination systemic chemotherapy using irinotecan and oxaliplatin for metastatic colorectal cancer now more easily achieve response rates previously obtained only with HAI therapy. Currently, HAI therapy should be only used as an adjunct to systemic chemotherapy, not as a replacement for systemic chemotherapy.

A strategy to improve the efficacy of HAI is to set up alternative treatments by infusing chemotherapy combinations thought to be more active than FUDR alone. In a recently published retrospective study, the impact of intrahepatic infusion of oxaliplatin with systemic FU/LV on patients with isolated unresectable liver metastases was investigated [22]. Most patients had synchronous (85%) and bilateral metastases (89%), and the median number of lesions was seven. Of the 87 patients, 69 (79%) were treated after failure of a first-line systemic chemotherapy. Twenty-three patients out of 87 (26%) were operated on and resection was performed in 21 (24%). Five-year overall survival was 56% in operated patients vs. none in the non-operated group.

6.2.4
Secondary Resectability Rates and Timing of Surgery

Secondary resectability rates following a response to preoperative chemotherapy have been evaluated in both retrospective and prospective studies (Table 6.1). One of the earliest reports on unresectable liver-only metastases treated with oxaliplatin-based chemotherapy, mostly with a chronomodulated regimen, showed a 38% secondary resection rate [23]. Conversely, when a larger cohort of unselected patients was considered, the same French group showed that the secondary resection rate was significantly inferior (12.5%) [24]. In phase II studies, almost similar, high resection rates (33% and 40%, respectively) were obtained with FOLFIRI and FOLFOX [25, 26]. The characteristics of patients included in these studies, in particular the extent of disease at diagnosis, may explain the difference in the secondary resection rates noted in the phase III trials. In the OPTIMOX-1 study, 620 patients not eligible for resection were treated with one of two first-line regimens of oxaliplatin plus FU/LV

(FOLFOX4 and "stop and go" FOLFOX7). Chemotherapy allowed resection in 101 patients (16%) [27]. In the study by Tournigand et al. [4], in which FOLFIRI followed by FOLFOX6 at progression was compared to the reverse sequence, secondary resectability rates favored FOLFOX in first-line therapy (22% vs. 9%). In a phase III study of 244 previously untreated patients, the triplet combination FOLFOXIRI conferred superior resection rates over FOLFIRI: 15% vs. 6% in the entire cohort and 36% vs. 12% in patients with liver-only metastases [8].

When biologic agents are added to cytotoxic chemotherapy, the likelihood of a salvage resection after tumor downsizing is increased. In the CRYSTAL study, overall and R0 resection rates were significantly higher for cetuximab + FOLFIRI than for FOLFIRI alone (6% vs. 2.5% and 4.3% vs. 1.5%, respectively). Not unexpectedly, higher rates of R0 resection were obtained in the subgroup of patients with disease confined to the liver (9.8% vs. 4.5%) [11. Similarly, the OPUS study, in which cetuximab was associated to FOLFOX, showed improved resectability rates in the arm of patients treated with the biologic (overall: 6.5% vs. 3.6%; R0: 4.7% vs. 2.4%) [12]. Higher rates of salvage resection were recently reported in the CELIM study for both cetuximab plus FOLFOX (38%) and cetuximab plus FOLFIRI (30%) [13]. However, the study included patients with liver-only unresectable metastases, although a retrospective critical review showed that 32% of the patients had resectable disease at baseline.

Similar results have been obtained with the use of bevacizumab. A retrospective analysis of data of the NO16966 study showed that bevacizumab in combination with oxaliplatin-based chemotherapy increased the rates of curative intent surgery in all patients (8.4% vs. 6.1%) and in those whose metastatic disease was confined to the liver (19.2% vs. 12.9%) [15]. Similar rates (10.4% and 20.3%, respectively) were reported for the combination bevacizumab-oxaliplatin in the BEAT study, which also yielded comparable results when bevacizumab was administered with irinotecan (6.5% in the entire population and 14.3% in patients with liver-only metastases) [28] (Table 6.1). Recently, in a multicenter phase II study involving patients with unresectable liver-only disease, bevacizumab in combination with oxaliplatin and capecitabine achieved a 32% conversion to resectable disease [16].

Collectively, theses results are undoubtedly promising. Nevertheless, there still is a wide range of secondary resection rates that may be related to different selection criteria for patient inclusion into different studies. In fact, the definition of unresectability varies significantly between studies, leading in some cases to the inclusion of patients with "not optimally resectable" disease. Therefore, data on resectability are not easily comparable.

In responding patients, an area of controversy is whether to treat them until the "maximal effect" is reached or to discontinue chemotherapy once the disease has been reduced to the point at which hepatic resection is feasible. As a general rule, preoperative chemotherapy should be stopped as soon as the disease becomes resectable. In fact, the policy of pursuing the "maximal effect" has many potential disadvantages. Firstly, maximal shrinking might be associated with a complete radiologic response of one or more hepatic lesions, a fact that may render surgery nonfeasible (see the section "Disappeared Liver Metastases"). Secondly, prolonging chemotherapy may have detrimental effects on the hepatic parenchyma. Data indicate that the rate of postoperative complications or hepatic insufficiency is strictly dependent on the duration of preoperative treatment, with the greatest increase after 6–9 cycles [29, 30]. Finally, in most circumstances the definition of the "maximal effect" is made *a posteriori*, when the re-growth of liver metastases is observed at re-staging. This situation is similar to that of patients progressing while on chemotherapy, which will be discussed in detail further below.

6.2.5
Results of Surgery in Patients with Secondary Resectable Disease

Bismuth et al. [31] were the first to demonstrate that some responding patients with extensive liver disease could undergo radical resection after chemotherapy and that long-term survival could be achieved. After this seminal report, in 2004 the authors reported on their updated series of 1439 patients managed over 11 years, of whom 1104 had initially unresectable disease [32]. After a mean of ten courses of mostly oxaliplatin-based chemotherapy, 138 patients (12.5%) achieved a sufficient response to permit secondary curative hepatic resection (Table 6.1); 75% of the resections were major hepatectomies and 93% were potentially curative (R0). Postoperative morbidity and 60-day mortality rates were 28% and 0.7%, respectively. The median survival and 5- and 10-year survival rates were 39 months, 33% and 23%, respectively. Although not as good as those of patients who underwent primary surgery without chemotherapy, these results were impressive. Other studies have shown survival rates ranging from 37% to 58% at 5 years [23, 33-34]. While prolonged survival can be expected, the question remains whether in such patients the intent of hepatic resection can properly be termed "curative," since cure is rarely achieved. In fact, reports indicate that in the vast majority of patients undergoing hepatic resection after neoadjuvant chemotherapy the disease recurs. We reported our experience with 34 out of 104 (32.7%) patients with initially unresectable disease that, following neoadjuvant oxaliplatin-based chemotherapy, was converted, during the years 2000–2003, to a resectable situation [35]. While the 3-year OS of these patients resembled that obtained in 116 patients who underwent resection upfront, the 3-year disease-free survival (DFS) was significantly inferior (21% vs. 50.5%). In fact, the disease recurred in almost all patients (94%), usually soon after liver resection (median DFS 8.7 months) and with an increased frequency of extrahepatic localizations, either alone or associated with a hepatic recurrence. Different results were obtained by Adam et al. [36]. The authors analyzed 148 patients with initially unresectable disease who underwent rescue surgery, with a minimum follow-up of 5 years. OS and DFS 5- and 10-year survival rates were 33%, 27% and 19%, 27%, respectively. In 76% of patients, the disease recurred, with a pattern slightly different from that observed in our study: while the intrahepatic recurrence rate was similar, the proportion of isolated extrahepatic recurrences was significantly inferior. Sixteen percent of patients were considered cured (i.e., without recurrence after 5 years from the last resection), albeit cure was obtained in one third of patients after reiterate resections of intra- or extrahepatic recurrences. The major drawback of this study is that it included patients operated on over a long period (1988–2002), thus questioning whether patients considered in the early 1990s to have unresectable disease would still have been evaluated as such in 2010. While further study is needed to clarify the outcome of these patients, the results published so far strongly support the policy of offering liver surgery to all patients whose metastases are sufficiently downsized by chemotherapy.

6.3
Resectable Liver Metastases

6.3.1
Rationale

Surgical resection is the mainstay of the treatment of hepatic colorectal metastases. However, it is still considered only a "potentially" curative treatment since, even after successful hepatic resection, the majority of patients suffer disease recurrence. Preoperative therapy has been repeatedly shown to be effective and safe in several types of solid tumors, such as rectal and esophageal carcinomas, prompting an evolution of the modern treatment of gastrointestinal tract cancers towards a multimodal approach.

The efficacy of the newer regimens has expanded the use of chemotherapy in patients with initially resectable disease because of several theoretical advantages. Firstly, it is possible to test chemoresponsiveness. The opportunity to demonstrate regimen-specific efficacy is useful to determine whether a treatment should be given postoperatively, thus avoiding ineffective chemotherapy. One might argue that progression during chemotherapy could render the tumor unresectable, whereas otherwise resection would have offered a potentially curative treatment. However, it has been shown that primary resistance to chemotherapy associated with tumor progression is infrequent (~7%), with one third of these patients still eligible for hepatic resection [37]. Yet, cohort data suggest that tumor progression during chemotherapy predicts poor outcome after resection. In a study by Adam et al. [38], patients with multiple colorectal liver metastases whose tumors progressed during chemotherapy had a 5-year survival rate of only 8%, compared to 37% in those whose tumors responded to chemotherapy. Tumor progression may therefore be considered a proxy of an aggressive tumor biology whose natural course might not be influenced by hepatic resection. In fact, in that study, almost all patients (94%) experienced early tumor recurrence. Although the attitude of most surgeons to consider hepatic resection contraindicated in the presence of progressive disease can be criticized, it prevents unnecessary surgery or allows these patients to be treated with second-line agents to reassess tumor response. Secondly, a preoperative systemic approach can, in theory, eliminate micrometastatic deposits within and outside the liver. Thirdly, it may facilitate and allow a technically simpler liver resection by decreasing the magnitude of resection needed. This has been shown to be a key factor for reducing post-operative morbidity. Likewise, compared with immediate resection, it may reduce the rate of positive margins and limit the morbidity arising from unnecessary interventions by facilitating the identification of patients who are appropriate candidates for subsequent surgery. This was shown in the EORTC Intergroup trial 40983, in which a significant reduction in the rate of unnecessary laparotomy, from 11% to 5%, in patients treated with preoperative chemotherapy, was observed [37]. Fourthly, pathologic assessment of the response to chemotherapy may provide a more reliable stratification of patients' prognosis and serve as selection criterion for adjuvant therapies. In a report from the Mayo Clinic, when the three most often used clinical scoring systems (the Fong, Nordlinger, and Iwatsuki scores) were used to evaluate 662 patients who underwent resection for colorectal liver metastases, none of the scoring systems were found to be predictive of survival or recurrence [39]. By contrast, histological tumor regression, graded by the extent of fibrosis and the presence of residual tumor cells, is emerging as a powerful prognostic tool and surrogate marker of tumor biology. In the study of Blazer et al. [40], response to preoperative systemic therapy was the only independent predictor of survival after hepatic resection, along with margin status. Of note, although further investigations are needed, the data thus far indicate that the extent of tumor regression is independent of the duration of chemotherapy [30, 41]. Therefore, a short course of preoperative chemotherapy might retain all the "survival" advantages while reducing the possible detrimental effects. Moreover, preoperative treatment ensures that all patients are treated, in contrast to postoperative chemotherapy. In the EORTC trial, > 30% of patients did not receive any adjuvant treatment, approximately 20% stopped postoperative chemotherapy after 1–3 cycles, and 60% had a dose reduction or delayed cycle administration. Finally, preoperative chemotherapy has the potential to improve survival.

Despite these benefits, there is still no universal agreement amongst treating surgeons and medical oncologists whether to give neoadjuvant chemotherapy prior to hepatectomy in patients with resectable disease, due in part to the question of the oncologic benefits and to the well-known drawbacks, including hepatic toxicity and the likelihood of inducing a complete radiologic response, which may render inoperable some patients with initially resectable liver metastases because of the absence of visible residual tumor.

6.3.2
Results

Several retrospective studies have demonstrated that preoperative chemotherapy increases curative resection rates, enables more conservative surgery, and permits the tailoring of postoperative chemotherapy based on the preoperative response. In addition, cohort analyses demonstrated that, in patients who were objective responders, prolonged survival can be obtained [40, 42, 43]. A single-center, non-randomized study published by Gruenberger et al. [44] showed that preoperative treatment with six cycles of XELOX or FOLFOX in 50 patients with potentially curable metastatic colorectal cancer obtained a 73% response rate and a R0 surgery rate of 93%. The median recurrence-free survival was significantly better in patients with tumor response (24.7 months) than in patients with stable disease (8.2 months) or tumor progression (3 months). A recent systematic review of all published series on the use of preoperative systemic chemotherapy prior to hepatectomy in patients with resectable disease [23 studies (3278 patients): 1 phase III randomized control trial (level I), 3 phase II studies (level II), and 19 observational studies (level III)] showed that tumor progression was detected in 15% of the patients, a rate that is almost two-fold higher than the rate reported in the EORTC trial 40983 [37, 45]. From this review analysis, however, it is not possible to quantify the proportion of patients in whom progression precluded surgery. Nordlinger et al. [37] reported that in the EORTC trial 40983 66% of patients with progressive disease could not undergo hepatic resection; yet, in 50% of these patients progression was outside the liver, suggesting that they would have received unnecessary liver surgery if they had been operated on immediately. The above-mentioned review analysis included other interesting data. Firstly, the median rate of complete resection with clear margins on histological examination (R0 resection) was 93%. Secondly, liver surgery after a limited course of chemotherapy (the median number of cycles was 6) was shown to be safe. In fact, median perioperative mortality and morbidity (all complications) rates were 2% and 27%, thus comparing favorably with the rates obtained after upfront resection when considering that almost 70% of patients underwent major hepatectomies.

The most disputed issue remains the oncologic benefit. Few retrospective studies have shown that preoperative chemotherapy significantly prolongs OS in high-risk patients. In a small series of 71 patients with multiple (≥ 5) resectable colorectal liver metastases, Tanaka et al. [46] demonstrated that preoperative chemotherapy was an independent predictor of OS, with a striking difference in 5-year survival estimates between individuals who did and those who did not receive preoperative chemotherapy (38.9% vs. 20.7%, respectively). In patients with synchronous liver metastases undergoing delayed hepatic resection after preoperative chemotherapy, Allen et al. [47] obtained 5-year survival rates of 87% in those patients whose tumors did not progress during chemotherapy. Therefore, we and others have begun to use preoperative chemotherapy in selected patients at high risk for early recurrence and reduced survival, such as those with more than three synchronous liver metastases [48, 49]. More recently, many centers have progressively expanded their indications for a multimodality approach to include almost all patients with initially resectable metastases. However, at present, the demonstration of a clear survival advantage from preoperative chemotherapy still requires level I evidence. In fact, the only available randomized trial (EORTC trial 40983) investigated the use of perioperative chemotherapy [37] and it remains unknown whether the positive effects reported in the treatment arm were related to preoperative or postoperative therapy. Nonetheless, intriguing information can be obtained from this trial. The study randomly assigned patients with resectable disease and a maximum of four liver metastases to perioperative chemotherapy (FOLFOX4: six cycles before and six cycles after surgery) or first-line surgery and observation. The primary end-point was increased PFS. After a median follow-up of 3.9 years, the absolute increase in 3-year PFS rate with the addition of perioperative chemotherapy was 7.3% (from 28.1% to 35.4%) in all eligible patients, which further increased to 9.2% (from 33.2% to 42.4%) in patients who had resection; although this endpoint was not prespecified, the increase was significant. The initial report did not prove a positive effect of perioperative chemotherapy on PFS, but the authors recently updated their results (ASCO 2009), showing a significant increase in PFS in an intent-to-treat analysis of all randomized patients. In addition, while almost 90% of patients had a full course of preoperative chemotherapy, approximately 50% of patients either did not receive postoperative chemotherapy (30%) or had a very short course (~20%). Therefore, it might be inferred that the survival advantage was due to the preoperative chemotherapy. By contrast, Reddy et al. [50] demonstrated in a cohort of 499 patients with initially resectable synchronous liver metastases that post-hepatectomy chemotherapy was an independent determinant of both OS and DFS while preoperative chemotherapy was not. In particular, OS figures according to the time of chemotherapy administration were as follows: no chemotherapy, median 36 months; prehepatectomy chemotherapy, median 53 months; post-hepatectomy chemotherapy, median 76 months; and perioperative chemotherapy, median 67 months. This result was further confirmed in a subset analysis of low-risk patients without extrahepatic disease, less than three metastases, and in whom concurrent ablation was not required for tumor clearance. Similarly, we recently showed that in patients with solitary metachronous liver metastases of < 5 cm, preoperative chemotherapy did not confer a survival advantage [51].

6.3.3
Strategy Proposal

The theoretical benefits of neoadjuvant chemotherapy have led many authors to systematically propose this treatment strategy. However, available studies have failed to demonstrate survival benefits from systematic neoadjuvant chemotherapy; indeed, some drawbacks have been reported, such as chemotherapy-related liver damage and tumor disappearance. Further studies are needed to establish shared guidelines as the policies of different surgical centers vary extremely. According to our experience and that obtained in published studies, despite their low level of evidence, some indications for neoadjuvant chemotherapy may be suggested:
- More than three metastases, both synchronous and metachronous.
- Associated extrahepatic disease, independent of the characteristics of the liver metastases.
- Risk of non-radical resection due to the site of metastasis and its relationship with intrahepatic vascular structures.

Immediate surgery is preferred in case of:
- Metachronous solitary metastasis.
- Risk of metastases disappearing.

In patients with up to three metastases, no recommendations can be made (except in the case of a metachronous solitary lesion). In our center, immediate resection is usually planned, but the final decision is based on a case-by case evaluation, considering the complete prognostic profile of the patient in a multidisciplinary setting. The synchronous presentation of metastases should not be considered an absolute indication for neoadjuvant chemotherapy.

This proposal represents an attempt to standardize treatment strategy for patients with liver metastases, but it awaits stronger evidence to guide practice.

6.4
Chemotherapy-related Liver Injuries

Although preoperative chemotherapy has many advantages, there has been growing concern about the potential for hepatic toxicities caused by the various systemic agents and regimens. Clinical data have shown associations between specific drugs and histological changes in the liver parenchyma. Worthy of note is the fact that, since patients are frequently treated with a combination of systemic agents, synergistic toxicity is likely. The types of pathology observed in liver specimens obtained from patients treated with preoperative chemotherapy can be classified in two categories: non-alcoholic fatty liver disease (NAFLD) and sinusoidal injury.

The broad spectrum of pathological states encompassed by NAFLD ranges from bland, non-progressive steatosis to steatohepatitis, advanced fibrosis, and cirrhosis. Steatosis, which denotes the pathologic accumulation of lipids within hepatocytes, is considered the earliest stage of NAFLD. It is classified as mild when < 30% of hepatocytes are affected by fatty infiltration, moderate with 30–60% fatty infiltration, and severe with > 60% (Fig. 6.2a). In later stages of the disease, steatosis is accompanied by an inflammatory response that defines steatohepatitis. The distinctive features of steatohepatitis include steatosis, monomorphic and neutrophilic portal and lobular inflammation, and perisinusoidal fibrosis in lobular zone 3 (Fig. 6.2b). Other common morphological features are hepatocellular ballooning, poorly formed Mallory's hyaline, and glycogenated nuclei. Steatohepatitis is assessed with the NAFLD Activity Score, which is the unweighted sum of the score for steatosis (0–3), lobular inflammation (0–3), and ballooning degeneration (0–2). A score ≥ 5 indicates the presence of steatohepatitis, whereas a score of 3–4 is regarded as borderline. While steatosis and steatohepatitis directly interfere with the function of hepatocytes, sinusoidal injury results from damage to the endothelial cells lining the sinusoids of the liver. This injury, termed sinusoidal obstruction syndrome, can lead to portal hypertension, ascites, hyperbilirubinemia, and, in severe cases, liver failure. One of the hallmarks of sinusoidal obstruction syndrome is sinusoidal dilation (Fig. 6.2c, d).

In the following, the association between preoperative chemotherapy and these pathologic findings and their clinical implications in patients undergoing liver resection are summarized.

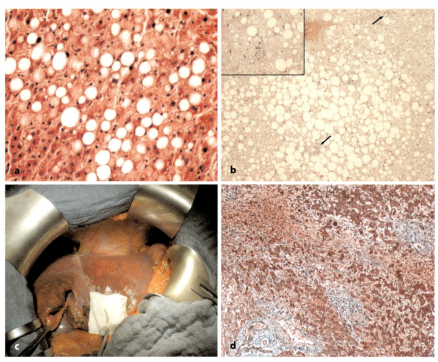

Fig. 6.2 Spectrum of chemotherapy-associated liver injury. **a** Moderate macrovesicular steatosis: approximately 40% of hepatocytes are distended by large fat droplets. **b** Steatohepatitis: various degrees of inflammation can be seen scattered throughout the lobule (*arrows*) in a background of marked steatosis (> 60%). The *insert* shows a magnification (× 40) of an inflammatory focus. **c** Macroscopic aspect of the liver, with oxaliplatin-associated injury ("blue" liver). **d** Microscopic demonstration of sinusoidal distension in the centrilobular region (hematoxylin and eosin, magnification × 200)

6.4.1
Chemotherapy and Steatosis

An association between steatosis and chemotherapy was first described in the early 1990s, in patients treated with FU. Radiographic evidence of steatosis was seen in 30-47% of these patients. More recently, it was demonstrated that all of the chemotherapy agents used in colorectal cancer are capable of causing steatosis [52]. Due to the potential of steatosis to directly interfere with the function of hepatocytes, several studies have examined its impact on patient outcome following resection. In most series, higher rates of postoperative complications (30–62%) were observed. Specifically, the data indicate that in patients with moderate to severe steatosis (i.e., > 30%) there is a greater likelihood of transfusion and an increased risk of postoperative liver insufficiency, biliary leakage, infectious complications, and longer mean intensive care unit stay [53-55]. McCormack et al. [56] also noted a non-statistically significant trend toward higher mortality, which was not confirmed in other surgical series. However, in most studies, steatosis was not differentiated from steatohepatitis as a separate pathological entity. In a study by Vauthey et al. [52], simple steatosis without inflammation was not associated with increased postoperative morbidity or mortality.

6.4.2
Irinotecan and Steatohepatitis

Steatohepatitis was first observed as a complication of chemotherapy in a small surgical series reported by Fernandez et al. [57], who noted that 12 out of 14 patients with steatohepatitis had received irinotecan. The association between irinotecan and steatohepatitis was clearly demonstrated in a large bi-institutional study from our center and the M.D. Anderson Cancer Center [52]. According to the results of that study, overall, 20% of patients receiving irinotecan developed steatohepatitis independent of BMI, although the risk was higher in patients with BMI >25 kg/m^2 (25% vs. 12%). A trend toward a higher risk for steatohepatitis in obese patients was also reported in other series. Unlike simple steatosis, irinotecan-induced steatohepatitis appears to have clinically relevant consequences. In fact, we reported a significantly higher 90-day mortality (14.7%) in patients with steatohepatitis than in those without (1.6%); in addition, mortality was mostly related to the risk of developing end-stage liver failure. Other groups have reported similarly adverse outcomes in patients with steatohepatitis [57, 58]. Given this finding, caution is recommended in obese patients treated with preoperative irinotecan, especially when the planned resection is a major hepatectomy.

6.4.3
Oxaliplatin and Sinusoidal Dilation

Oxaliplatin's major liver toxicity appears to be directed against the endothelial cells lining the sinusoids. In a retrospective case study, Rubbia-Brandt et al. [59] found that 78% of patients treated with oxaliplatin developed sinusoidal dilation, which is graded semiquantitatively according to the extent of centrilobular involvement (grades 0–3). Similarly, we reported that oxaliplatin was associated with high rates of moderate to severe (grades 2–3) sinusoidal injury (19% vs. 2% in patients who did not receive chemotherapy) [52], a finding consistently confirmed in other studies [60-62]. In addition, ongoing analysis has shown that oxaliplatin is associated with a broader pattern of parenchymal hepatic injury, including nodular regenerative hyperplasia, peliosis, and centrilobular vein fibrosis [63]. The clinical implications of these complications remain to be fully evaluated. Although overt liver failure in patients with oxaliplatin-induced sinusoidal obstruction syndrome has rarely been reported, a number of case reports have described the development of portal hypertensive sequelae, such as ascites and variceal bleeding. Recently, Overman et al. [64]

found that oxaliplatin-based chemotherapy induced spleen size enlargement in 86% of patients, with a > 50% volume increase from baseline in 24% of the individuals studied (Fig. 6.3a). The increase in spleen size, which correlates with the cumulative oxaliplatin dose (Fig. 6.3b), exposes patients to the risk of prolonged thrombocytopenia in the first year after completion of chemotherapy, especially those with splenic enlargement > 50%. Noteworthy is the observation that increases in spleen size correlate with increasing grade of hepatic sinusoidal dilation (Fig. 6.3c) and,

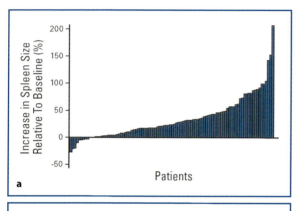

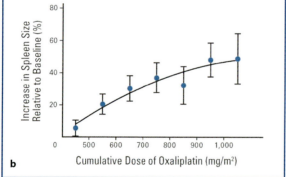

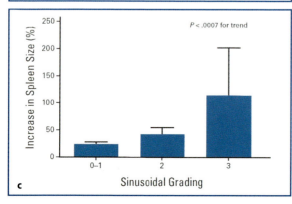

Fig. 6.3 a Changes in spleen size in 135 patients treated in the adjuvant or neoadjuvant setting and (**b**) its correlation with cumulative oxaliplatin dosage. **c** Increases in spleen size significantly correlate with histopathologic grade of sinusoidal injury. (From [64], reprinted with permission. ©2008 American Society of Clinical oncology. All rights reserved)

thus, can serve as a simple method for identifying patients at risk for this toxicity. From a surgical standpoint, the strongest evidence that oxaliplatin increases surgical morbidity comes from the EORTC trial 40983, in which patients who received perioperative oxaliplatin-based chemotherapy had a higher incidence of complications (25%) than did patients who had surgery alone (16%). Yet, there was no difference in mortality between the two groups. The observation that oxaliplatin increases surgical morbidity but not mortality has been reported in other studies [65-67]. Aloia et al. [65] found that patients treated with preoperative chemotherapy, mostly oxaliplatin, tended to have a higher rate of morbidity than patients who were resected upfront. Upon further analysis, the authors demonstrated that individuals with severe vascular changes had a greater need for blood transfusions than did those without injury. Conversely, several other case series, including ours, showed no difference in morbidity or mortality [52, 61, 68]. As previously mentioned, reports indicate a direct correlation between the number of preoperative chemotherapy cycles and morbidity rates, which significantly increase after six courses of chemotherapy [29, 67].

An obvious concern is that treatments in which oxaliplatin is associated with irinotecan could lead to greater toxicity. However, so far the data are scarce. A pooled analysis of postoperative results of patients who underwent hepatic resection after FOLFOXIRI chemotherapy in phase II/III trials indicated a surgical complication rate of 27%, with no mortality [69]. In terms of pathologic changes, sinusoidal dilation was noted in 100% of the patients (all were grade 1–2) and steatohepatitis in 4%.

6.4.4
Bevacizumab

Bevacizumab, as a potent inhibitor of angiogenesis, has the potential to adversely affect liver regeneration, increase bleeding, and impair wound healing. This last concern was raised as a result of a pooled analysis of two large clinical trials showing that patients who underwent any surgery while being treated with bevacizumab had a higher rate (13% vs. 3.4%) of grade III/IV wound-healing complications than patients treated with placebo [70]. Nonetheless, data are emerging on the safety of hepatectomy after bevacizumab administration. Kesmodel et al. [71] compared the outcomes of 81 patients who received preoperative bevacizumab-containing regimens with those of 44 patients who received chemotherapy alone and found no difference in morbidity or mortality between the two groups. Similar results were obtained by others [72, 73] but there is still concern, corroborated by the fact that bevacizumab is slowly cleared from the body and has a median half-life of 20 days. Therefore, an important consideration is how long prior to surgery should bevacizumab be stopped. While some authors found that the time interval between bevacizumab and surgery did not influence the complication rate, others noted a trend, although not statistically significant, toward more hepatic complications when bevacizumab was given within 8 weeks prior to surgery. A general agreement has been reached in considering surgery safe when performed 6–8 weeks after the last administration of bevacizumab. Therefore, one practical rule might be to avoid administering bevacizumab during the last chemotherapy cycle.

One of the most intriguing findings is the observation that bevacizumab may protect against sinusoidal damage. This protective benefit of bevacizumab was first seen by Ribero et al. [74], who showed that patients treated with bevacizumab had a significantly lower incidence and severity of sinusoidal injury. To date, there is no indication whether the severe parenchymal lesions associated with oxaliplatin, such as nodular regenerative hyperplasia and those associated with sinusoidal obstruction syndrome, are reversible with bevacizumab.

6.4.5
Cetuximab

Preclinical data are mixed regarding the effect of EGFR inhibition on hepatic regeneration. Whereas one report presented strong genetic evidence that EGFR is essential in hepatic regeneration, another showed that cetuximab administration does not adversely affect hepatectomized mice. In the clinical setting, there are relatively few data available regarding the safety of administering cetuximab prior to hepatectomy. In a series by Adam et al. [75], patients with first-line chemotherapy-resistant tumors were treated with cetuximab-containing second-line chemotherapy. Of the 151 patients with initially unresectable disease, 27 obtained tumor downsizing and underwent subsequent hepatic resection. Postoperative 60-day mortality was 3.7% (the only patient who died succumbed to liver failure following a repeat major hepatectomy), with a complication rate of 50%. Histopathologic liver abnormalities were found in nine patients (36%), without specific lesions attributable to cetuximab.

6.5
Disappeared Liver Metastases

Although rare, complete pathologic disappearance of all liver metastases after chemotherapy is associated with considerable OS and is a strong predictor of both prolonged survival and disease cure. However, complete clinical response (CCR) of colorectal metastases according to RECIST criteria has been shown to be of limited predictive value for complete pathologic response (CPR) and disease cure. Adam et al. [76] observed CPR in 4% of patients undergoing resection following preoperative chemotherapy; none of these patients had CCR. Recent progresses in systemic and intra-arterial chemotherapy has resulted in the disappearance of some liver metastases on liver imaging (up to 9% of patients). It now appears that conventional imaging, particularly positron emission tomography (PET) and computed tomography (CT) scans, is less accurate after treatment than in untreated patients. Two recent studies showed that the sensitivity of contrast-enhanced CT in detecting metastases after chemotherapy is 65–70%, while ^{18}F-fluoro-2-deoxy-D-glucose (FDG)-PET has a sensitivity of 49–62%, significantly lower than the expected results with CT and PET in unselected patients. After prolonged chemotherapy, the liver parenchyma changes, becoming steatotic. At the same time, this efficient chemotherapy reduces the size of the liver metastases but also modifies their echogenicity on ultrasound (US) and their density on CT. Consequently, it is increasingly the case that some small-sized liver metastases disappear regardless of the preoperative imaging technique, i.e., US, CT, PET, or magnetic resonance imaging (MRI). Considering the absence of any reliable preoperative tool to assess CPR, only surgical resection with concomitant pathologic examination of the specimen enables a definitive diagnosis. In addition, the complete disappearance of metastases on imaging should not contraindicate surgery, since a majority of these patients will not have a CPR.

Elias et al. [77], in their first series, identified 54 disappeared liver metastases (DLM) in 15 patients. In four patients (27%), the liver metastases were identified and resected at laparotomy. Of the remaining 11 patients, liver metastases in three relapsed during the follow-up (20%), while in eight patients (53%) there was no recurrence after a median follow-up of 31 months. In a more recent series from the same institution, 69 DLM (16 patients) were left in situ after surgical exploration. During a mean follow-up of 51 months, they did not reappear in 10 patients (62%) [78]. By contrast, Benoist et al. [79] evaluated 66 liver metastases that disappeared during chemotherapy in 38 patients and observed macroscopic persistence at laparotomy in 20 DLM (30%), microscopic residual disease in 12 of 15 DLM (18%), and early in situ recurrence in 23 of 31 DLM (35%). Overall residual cancer was observed in 83% of the DLM. In a recent paper, Tanaka et al. [80] analyzed 86 DLM in 23 patients who received preoperative chemotherapy and underwent hepatectomy: 31 DLM were found at laparotomy (36%). Persistent microscopic residual disease or recurrence in situ was observed in 30.6% of the liver metastases with a complete response on preoperative imaging. Similar data were recently reported by Auer et al. [81], who assessed 118 DLM in 39 patients who had undergone chemotherapy before hepatic resection: 68 metastases were resected but only 11% were detected during the laparotomy, and 50 were followed clinically. The rate of persistent disease was 36%. Overall, the true complete response rate among DLM was 75 of 118 (64%), including 44 complete responses (59%) confirmed by pathologic assessment and 31 (41%) confirmed by clinical follow-up. The authors also showed that normalization of the CEA level after chemotherapy, inability to detect the lesion by MRI, and the use of intra-arterial chemotherapy were independently associated with a true CPR at multivariate analysis. In our series of 171 patients treated by resection after preoperative chemotherapy between January 2004 and December 2009, 10.3% of the patients had one or more DLM on all preoperative imaging techniques (67 DLM in 33 patients). However, 67% of DLM were found intraoperatively, either with a simple liver inspection or, most frequently (86% of the cases), with the use of intraoperative ultrasound (IOUS). By combining pathologic data on residual viable tumor cells and follow-up data on in situ recurrences for those lesions left untreated at the time of operation, we found that two-thirds of the DLM were not cured (persistent disease rate of 61.2%, unpublished data). Therefore, in patients with DLM, resection of the sites of metastases is mandatory when clearly identified with the use of IOUS. Conversely, in those 30–70% of patients in whom DLM cannot be identified at IOUS, with or without the use of an i.v. contrast agent, blind resection of the site is recommended when the hepatectomy can be easily performed. Observation might be the preferred choice in those lesions deeply located requiring a major hepatectomy that would not be performed to clear all other visible lesions.

References

1. Saltz LB, Cox JV, Blanke C et al (2000) Irinotecan plus fluorouracil and leucovorin for metastatic colorectal cancer. Irinotecan Study Group. N Engl J Med 343:905-914
2. Douillard JY, Cunningham D, Roth AD et al (2000) Irinotecan combined with fluorouracil compared with fluorouracil alone as first-line treatment for metastatic colorectal cancer: A multicentre randomised trial. Lancet 355:1041-1047
3. Goldberg RM, Sargent DJ, Morton RF et al (2004) A randomized controlled trial of fluorouracil plus leucovorin, irinotecan, and oxaliplatin combinations in patients with previously untreated metastatic colorectal cancer. J Clin Oncol 22:23-30
4. Tournigand C, André T, Achille E et al (2004) FOLFIRI followed by FOLFOX6 or the reverse sequence in advanced colorectal cancer: a randomized GERCOR study. J Clin Oncol 22:229-237
5. Kohne CH, van Cutsem E, Wils J et al (2005) Phase III study of weekly high-dose infusional fluorouracil plus folinic acid with or without irinotecan in patients with metastatic colorectal cancer: European Organisation for Research and Treatment of Cancer Gastrointestinal Group Study 40986. J Clin Oncol 23:4856-4865
6. Giacchetti S, Perpoint B, Zidani R et al (2000) Phase III multicenter randomized trial of oxaliplatin added to chronomodulated fluorouracil-leucovorin as first-line treatment of metastatic colorectal cancer. J Clin Oncol 18:136-147
7. Grothey A, Sargent D, Goldberg RM et al (2004) Survival of patients with advanced colorectal cancer improves with the availability of fluorouracil-leucovorin, irinotecan, and oxaliplatin in the course of treatment. J Clin Oncol 22:1209-1214
8. Falcone A, Ricci S, Brunetti I et al (2007) Phase III trial of infusional fluorouracil, leucovorin, oxaliplatin, and irinotecan (FOLFOXIRI) compared with infusional fluorouracil, leucovorin, and irinotecan (FOLFIRI) as first-line treatment for metastatic colorectal cancer: the Gruppo Oncologico Nord Ovest. J Clin Oncol 25:1670-1676
9. Arkenau HT, Arnold D, Cassidy J et al (2008) Efficacy of oxaliplatin plus capecitabine or infusional fluorouracil/leucovorin in patients with metastatic colorectal cancer: a pooled analysis of randomized trials. J Clin Oncol 26:5910-5917
10. Folprecht G, Grothey A, Alberts S et al (2005) Neoadjuvant treatment of unresectable colorectal liver metastases: correlation between tumour response and resection rates. Ann Oncol 16:1311-1319
11 Van Cutsem E, Köhne CH, Hitre E et al (2009) Cetuximab and chemotherapy as initial treatment for metastatic colorectal cancer. N Engl J Med 360:1408-1417
12. Bokemeyer C, Bondarenko I, Makhson A et al (2009) Fluorouracil, leucovorin, and oxaliplatin with and without cetuximab in the first-line treatment of metastatic colorectal cancer. J Clin Oncol 27:663-667
13. Folprecht G, Gruenberger T, Bechstein WO et al (2010) Tumour response and secondary resectability of colorectal liver metastases following neoadjuvant chemotherapy with cetuximab: the CELIM randomised phase 2 trial. Lancet Oncol 11:38-47

14. Hurwitz H, Fehrenbacher L, Novotny W et al (2004) Bevacizumab plus irinotecan, fluorouracil, and leucovorin for metastatic colorectal cancer. N Engl J Med 350:2335-2342
15. Saltz LB, Clarke S, Diaz-Rubio E et al (2008) Bevacizumab in combination with oxaliplatin-based chemotherapy as first-line therapy in metastatic colorectal cancer: a randomized phase III study. J Clin Oncol 26:2013-2019
16. Wong R, Saffery C, Barbachano Y et al (2009) BOXER: A multicenter phase II trial of capecitabine and oxaliplatin plus bevacizumab as neoadjuvant treatment for patients with liver-only metastases from colorectal cancer unsuitable for upfront resection. Eur J Cancer 7(suppl):6076
17. Masi G, Vasile E, Loupakis F et al (2009) Bevacizumab (BV) in combination with FOLFOXIRI (irinotecan, oxaliplatin and infusional 5FU/LV) as first-line treatment of metastatic colorectal cancer (mCRC): a phase II study by the G.O.N.O. group. Ann Oncol 20 (Suppl 7)
18. Cohen AD, Kemeny NE (2003) An update on hepatic arterial infusion chemotherapy for colorectal cancer. Oncologist 8:553-566
19. Barber FD, Mavligit G, Kurzrock R (2004) Hepatic arterial infusion chemotherapy for metastatic colorectal cancer: a concise overview. Cancer Treat Rev 30:425-436
20. Meta-Analysis Group in Cancer (1996) Reappraisal of hepatic arterial infusion in the treatment of nonresectable liver metastases from colorectal cancer. Meta-Analysis Group in Cancer. J Nat Cancer Inst 88:223-224
21. Kerr DJ, McArdle CS, Ledermann J et al (2003) Intrahepatic arterial versus intravenous fluorouracil and folinic acid for colorectal cancer liver metastases: a multicentre randomised trial. Lancet 361:368-373
22. Goere D, Deshaies I, de Baere T et al (2010) Prolonged survival of initially unresectable hepatic colorectal cancer patients treated with hepatic arterial infusion of oxaliplatin followed by radical surgery of metastases. Ann Surg 251:686–691
23. Giacchetti S, Itzhaki M, Gruia G et al (1999) Long-term survival of patients with unresectable colorectal cancer liver metastases following infusional chemotherapy with 5-fluorouracil, leucovorin, oxaliplatin and surgery. Ann Oncol.10:663-669
24. Adam R, Delvart V, Pascal G et al (2004) Rescue surgery for unresectable colorectal liver metastases downstaged by chemotherapy: a model to predict long-term survival. Ann Surg 240:644-657
25. Barone C, Nuzzo G, Cassano A et al (2007) Final analysis of colorectal cancer patients treated with irinotecan and 5-fluorouracil plus folinic acid neoadjuvant chemotherapy for unresectable liver metastases. Br J Cancer 97:1035-1039
26. Alberts SR, Horvath WL, Maohoney MR et al (2005) Oxaliplatin, fluorouracil and leucovorin for patients with unresectable liver-only metastases from colorectal cancer: A North Central Cancer Treatment Group (NCCTG) phase II study. J Clin Oncol 23:1-7
27. Perez-Staub N, Lledo G, Paye F et al (2006) Surgery of colorectal metastasis in the Optimox 1 study. AGERCOR study. J Clin Oncol 24(18 suppl):3522
28. Van Cutsem E, Rivera F, Berry S et al (2009) Safety and efficacy of first-line bevacizumab with FOLFOX, XELOX, FOLFIRI and fluoropyrimidines in metastatic colorectal cancer: the BEAT study. Ann Oncol 20:1842-1847
29. Karoui M, Penna C, Amin-Hashem M et al (2006) Influence of preoperative chemotherapy on the risk of major hepatectomy for colorectal liver metastases. Ann Surg 243:1–7
30. Zorzi D, Kishi Y, Maru DM et al (2009) Extended preoperative chemotherapy does not improve pathologic response and increases postoperative liver insufficiency after hepatic resection for colorectal liver metastases (abstract 295). American society of clinical oncology 2009 Gastrointestinal Cancers Symposium, January 15–17, 2009, San Francisco, CA
31. Bismuth H, Adam R, Levi F et al (1996) Resection of nonresectable liver metastases from colorectal cancer after neoadjuvant chemotherapy. Ann Surg 224:509-522
32. Adam R, Delvart V, Pascal G et al (2004) Rescue surgery for unresectable colorectal liver metas-

tases downstaged by chemotherapy: a model to predict long-term survival. Ann Surg 240:644-657

33. Rivoire M, De Cian F, Meeus P et al (2002) Combination of neoadjuvant chemotherapy with cryotherapy and surgical resection for the treatment of unresectable liver metastases from colorectal carcinoma. Cancer 95:2283–2292

34. Masi G, Cupini S, Marcucci L et al (2006) Treatment with 5-fluorouracil/folinic acid, oxaliplatin, and irinotecan enables surgical resection of metastases in patients with initially unresectable metastatic colorectal cancer. Ann Surg Oncol 13:58-65

35. Capussotti L, Muratore M, Mulas MM et al (2006) Neoadjuvant chemotherapy and resection for initially irresectable colorectal liver metastases. Br J Surg 93:1001–1006

36. Adam R, Wicherts DA, de Haas RJ et al (2009) Patients with initially unresectable colorectal liver metastases: is there a possibility of cure? J Clin Oncol 27:1829-1835

37. Nordlinger B, Sorbye H, Glimelius B et al (2008) Perioperative chemotherapy with FOLFOX4 and surgery versus surgery alone for resectable liver metastases from colorectal cancer (EORTC Intergroup trial 40983): a randomised controlled trial. Lancet 371:1007-1016

38. Adam R, Pascal G, Castaing D et al (2004) Tumor progression while on chemotherapy. A contraindication to liver resection for multiple colorectal metastases? Ann Surg 240:1052–1064

39. Zakaria S, Donohue JH, Que FG et al (2007) Hepatic resection for colorectal metastases: value for risk scoring systems? Ann Surg 246:183-191

40. Blazer DG III, Kishi Y, Maru DM et al (2008) Pathologic response to preoperative chemotherapy: a new outcome end point after resection of hepatic colorectal metastases. J Clin Oncol 26:5344-5351

41. Ribero D, Wang H, Donadon M et al (2007) Bevacizumab improves pathologic response and protects against hepatic injury in patients treated with oxaliplatin- based chemotherapy for colorectal liver metastases. Cancer 110:2761–2767

42. Tanaka K, Adam R, Shimada H et al (2003) Role of neoadjuvant chemotherapy in the treatment of multiple colorectal metastases to the liver. Br J Surg 90:963–96

43. Allen PJ, Kemeny N, Jarnagin W et al (2003) Importance of response to neoadjuvant chemotherapy in patients undergoing resection of synchronous colorectal liver metastases. J Gastrointest Surg 7:109-115

44. Gruenberger B, Scheithauer W, Punzengruber R et al (2008) Importance of response to neoadjuvant chemotherapy in potentially curable colorectal cancer liver metastases. BMC Cancer 8:120

45. Chua TC, Saxena A, Liauw W et al (2010) Systematic review of randomized and nonrandomized trials of the clinical response and outcomes of neoadjuvant systemic chemotherapy for resectable colorectal liver metastases. Ann Surg Oncol 17:492-501

46. Tanaka K, Adam R, Shimada H et al (2003) Role of neoadjuvant chemotherapy in the treatment of multiple colorectal metastases to the liver. Br J Surg 90:963–969

47. Allen PJ, Kemeny N, Jarnagin W et al (2003) Importance of response to neoadjuvant chemotherapy in patients undergoing resection of synchronous colorectal liver metastases. J Gastrointest Surg 7:109-115

48. Capussotti L, Viganò L, Ferrero A et al (2007) Timing of resection of liver metastases synchronous to colorectal tumor: proposal of prognosis-based decisional model. Ann Surg Oncol 14:1143-1150

49. Minagawa M, Yamamoto J, Miwa S et al (2006) Selection criteria for simultaneous resection in patients with synchronous liver metastasis. Arch Surg 141:1006-1012

50. Reddy SK, Zorzi D, Lum YW et al (2009) Timing of Multimodality Therapy for Resectable Synchronous Colorectal Liver Metastases: A Retrospective Multi-Institutional Analysis. Ann Surg Oncol 16:1809-1819

51. Adam R, Delvart V, Gorden L et al (in press) Is perioperative chemotherapy useful for metachronous solitary colorectal liver metastases? Ann Surg

52. Vauthey JN, Pawlik TM, Ribero D et al (2006) Chemotherapy regimen predicts steatohepati-

tis and an increase in 90-day mortality after surgery for hepatic colorectal metastases. J Clin Oncol 24:2065–2072

53. Kooby DA, Fong Y, Suriawinata A et al (2003) Impact of steatosis on perioperative outcome following hepatic resection. J Gastrointest Surg 7:1034–44

54. Behrns KE, Tsiotos GG, DeSouza NF et al (1998) Hepatic steatosis as a potential risk factor for major hepatic resection. J Gastrointest Surg 2:292–298

55. Belghiti J, Hiramatsu K, Benoist S et al (2000) Seven hundred forty-seven hepatectomies in the 1990s: an update to evaluate the actual risk of liver resection. J AmColl Surg 191:38–46

56. McCormack L, Petrowsky H, Jochum W et al (2007) Hepatic steatosis is a risk factor for postoperative complications after major hepatectomy: A matched case-control study. Ann Surg 245:923-930

57. Fernandez FG, Ritter J, Goodwin JW et al (2005) Effect of steatohepatitis associated with irinotecan or oxaliplatin pretreatment on resectability of hepatic colorectal metastases. J Am Coll Surg 200:845–853

58. Sasaki M, Itatsu K, Minato H et al (2007) Flare-up of nonalcoholic steatohepatitis after hepatectomy resulted in hepatic failure in a patient with type 2 diabetes mellitus. Dig Dis Sci 52:3473–3476

59. Rubbia-Brandt L, Audard V, Sartoretti P et al (2004) Severe hepatic sinusoidal obstruction associated with oxaliplatin-based chemotherapy in patients with metastatic colorectal cancer. Ann Oncol 15:460–466

60. Rubbia-Brandt L, Giostra E, Brezault C et al (2007) Importance of histological tumor response assessment in predicting the outcome in patients with colorectal liver metastases treated with neo-adjuvant chemotherapy followed by liver surgery. Ann Oncol 18:299-304

61. Pawlik TM, Olino K, Gleisner AL et al (2007) Preoperative chemotherapy for colorectal liver metastases: Impact on hepatic histology and postoperative outcome. J Gastrointest Surg 11:860–868

62. Kandutsch S, Klinger M, Hacker S et al (2008) Patterns of hepatotoxicity after chemotherapy for colorectal cancer liver metastases. Eur J Surg Oncol 34:1231–1236

63. Rubbia-Brandt L, Lauwers GY, Wang H et al (2010) Sinusoidal obstruction syndrome and nodular regenerative hyperplasia are frequent oxaliplatin associated liver lesions and partially prevented by bevacizumab in patients with hepatic colorectal metastasis. Histopathology 56:430-439

64. Overman MJ, Maru DM, Charnsangavej C et al (2010) Oxaliplatin-mediated increase in spleen size as a biomarker for the development of hepatic sinusoidal injury. J Clin Oncol 28:2549-2555

65. Aloia T, Sebagh M, Plasse M et al (2006) Liver histology and surgical outcomes after preoperative chemotherapy with fluorouracil plus oxaliplatin in colorectal cancer liver metastases. J Clin Oncol 24:4983– 4990

66. Welsh FK, Tilney HS, Tekkis PP et al (2007) Safe liver resection following chemotherapy for colorectal metastases is a matter of timing. Br J Cancer 96:1037–1042

67. Nakano H, Oussoultzoglou E, Rosso E et al (2008) Sinusoidal injury increases morbidity after major hepatectomy in patients with colorectal liver metastases receiving preoperative chemotherapy. Ann Surg 247:118-124

68. Mehta NN, Ravikumar R, Coldham CA et al (2008) Effect of preoperative chemotherapy on liver resection for colorectal liver metastases. Eur J Surg Oncol 34:782–786

69. Masi G, Loupakis F, Pollina L et al (2009) Long-term outcome of initially unresectable metastatic colorectal cancer patients treated with 5-fluorouracil/leucovorin, oxaliplatin, and irinotecan (FOLFOXIRI) followed by radical surgery of metastases. Ann Surg 249:420-425

70. Scappaticci FA, Fehrenbacher L, Cartwright T et al (2005) Surgical wound healing complications in metastatic colorectal cancer patients treated with bevacizumab. J Surg Oncol 91:173–180

71. Kesmodel SB, Ellis LM, Lin E et al (2008) Preoperative bevacizumab does not significantly increase postoperative complication rates in patients undergoing hepatic surgery for colorectal cancer liver metastases. J Clin Oncol. 26:5254 –5260
72. D'Angelica M, Kornprat P, Gonen M et al (2007) Lack of evidence for increased operative morbidity after hepatectomy with perioperative use of bevacizumab: A matched case-control study. Ann Surg Oncol 14:759 –765
73. Reddy SK, Morse MA, Hurwitz HI et al (2008) Addition of bevacizumab to irinotecan-and oxaliplatin-based preoperative chemotherapy regimens does not increase morbidity after resection of colorectal liver metastases. J Am Coll Surg 206:96 –106
74. Ribero D, Wang H, Donadon M et al (2007) Bevacizumab improves pathologic response and protects against hepatic injury in patients treated with oxaliplatin- based chemotherapy for colorectal liver metastases. Cancer 110:2761–2767
75. Adam R, Aloia T, Levi F et al (2007) Hepatic resection after rescue cetuximab treatment for colorectal liver metastases previously refractory to conventional systemic therapy. J Clin Oncol 25:4593-602
76. Adam R, Wicherts DA, de Haas RJ et al (2008) Complete Pathologic Response After Preoperative Chemotherapy for Colorectal Liver Metastases: Myth or Reality? J Clin Oncol 26:1635-1641
77. Elias D, Youssef O, Sideris L et al (2004) Evolution of Missing Colorectal Liver Metastases Following Inductive Chemotherapy and Hepatectomy. J Surg Oncol 86:4–9
78. Elias D, Goere D, Boige V et al (2007) Outcome of Posthepatectomy-Missing Colorectal Liver Metastases after Complete Response to Chemotherapy: Impact of Adjuvant Intra-arterial Hepatic Oxaliplatin. Ann Surg Oncol 14:3188–3194
79. Benoist S, Brouquet A, Penna C et al (2006) Complete Response of Colorectal Liver Metastases After Chemotherapy: Does It Mean Cure? J Clin Oncol 24:3939-3945
80. Tanaka K, Takakura H, Takeda K et al (2009) Importance of Complete Pathologic Response to Prehepatectomy Chemotherapy in Treating Colorectal Cancer Metastases Ann Surg 250:935-942
81. Auer RC, White R, Kemeny NE et al (2010) Predictors of a True Complete Response Among Disappearing Liver Metastases From Colorectal Cancer After Chemotherapy. Cancer 116:1502-1509

Synchronous Colorectal Liver Metastases

7

Abstract Radical surgery is the gold standard in the treatment of synchronous colorectal liver metastases. It prolongs patient survival and is potentially curative in some cases. Simultaneous colorectal and liver resection can be safely performed if minor hepatectomy is planned, whereas for major hepatectomy the results of simultaneous resection are controversial. Neoadjuvant chemotherapy helps to better select candidates for surgery, but there is no evidence in favour of its systematic application. In selected patients, such as those with more than three metastases, neoadjuvant chemotherapy may be beneficial. In patients with unresectable synchronous liver metastases, chemotherapy is the treatment of choice. In asymptomatic patients, chemotherapy should be immediately started with the primary tumor still in place. The risk of occlusion is low, especially if modern chemotherapy regimens are administered. In case of symptomatic primary tumor, chemotherapy must be preceded by symptoms treatment. Endoscopic metallic stents may represent an effective alternative to surgery in the treatment of occlusive symptoms. A multidisciplinary approach is mandatory in patients with primary colorectal cancer and synchronous liver metastases in order to define the optimal treatment strategy, which must be tailored to every single patient.

7.1
Introduction

Among patients with primary colorectal cancer, 20–30% have liver metastases at diagnosis [1, 2] (Fig. 7.1); however, only 15–20% of these patients are resectable [1, 2]. In the large majority of patients, resection is not possible because of the extent of the liver disease and/or the presence of further metastatic deposits, especially pulmonary and peritoneal ones [1, 2]. The prognosis of patients with synchronous liver metastases is related more to the metastases than to the primary tumor [1].

L. Viganò (✉)
Division of Hepato-Bilio-Pancreatic and Digestive Surgery, Mauriziano "Umberto I" Hospital, Turin, Italy

Surgical Treatment of Colorectal Liver Metastases. Lorenzo Capussotti (Ed.)
© Springer-Verlag Italia 2011

101

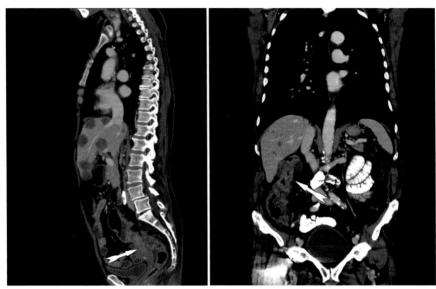

Fig. 7.1 Patients with primary colorectal cancer and synchronous liver metastases. Coronal images at CT scan. *Arrows* indicate primary tumor

The management of patients with colorectal cancer and synchronous liver metastases is complex since both the primary tumor and the metastatic disease have to be considered. A multidisciplinary approach is needed to correctly integrate all the required procedures, especially surgery and chemotherapy, but also endoscopic treatments and radiotherapy in selected cases. Different strategies have been proposed, as discussed in an increasing number of recently published papers; however, at present, neither evidence-based guidelines nor expert consensus are available. The majority of studies are retrospective monocenter series comprising a limited number of patients, with data collected across long time intervals.

This chapter considers the different management options for patients with synchronous liver metastases, with special attention paid to surgical indications, timing, and results. In order to adequately address these topics, patients with resectable and initially unresectable liver metastases are separately considered.

7.2
Resectable Synchronous Liver Metastases

At present, liver resection is the only potentially curative treatment of colorectal liver metastases [3-5]. Patients with synchronous metastases can also be scheduled for liver resection with curative intent. Even if in many surgical series synchronous metastases have been reported as a negative prognostic factor [2, 6, 7], liver surgery offers better survival results in comparison to palliative chemotherapy [8-16]. In the

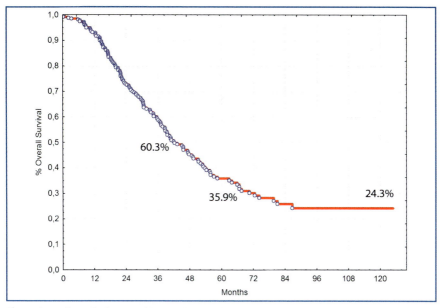

Fig. 7.2 Overall survival curve of 357 patients undergoing liver resection for synchronous colorectal metastases at the Hospital Mauriziano between January 1989 and January 2010

literature, 5-year survival rates after radical liver surgery range from 30 to 40% [8-16]. Between January 1989 and January 2010, 357 patients with synchronous liver metastases underwent hepatic resection at our hospital. After a median follow-up of 23.7 months, the 5-year survival rate was 35.9% (Fig. 7.2). Although high recurrence rates have been reported, in some cases surgery may even be curative. In a recent paper, our group reported an actual 10-year survival rate of 9.1% in 55 patients undergoing liver resection for synchronous liver metastases, i.e., five patients cured by surgery [7].

The optimal management of patients with resectable liver metastases synchronous to primary colorectal cancer is still controversial, with debate revolving around: (1) technical issues, i.e., the timing of colorectal and liver resection (simultaneous vs. delayed procedures); (2) oncologic issues, i.e., indications for neoadjuvant chemotherapy (systematic vs. in selected cases) and inclusion of radiotherapy in the treatment of rectal cancers.

7.2.1
Technical Issues

The timing of hepatic and colorectal surgery has been widely debated over the last decades and is still a matter of controversy. The pros and cons of both procedures have been reported, with the surgical strategy varying among the different centers.

Simultaneous resection presents the following advantages [9, 10, 17, 18]:

- The performance of only a single surgical procedure.
- The removal of all neoplastic foci and interruption of the "metastatic cascade".
- The avoidance of immunodepression after isolated primary tumor resection, which could enhance metastatic cell proliferation and allow tumor progression.

However, the following disadvantages of simultaneous resections have been discussed:

- The combination of a "clean" and a "contaminated" surgical procedure and thus the higher risk of septic complications, which could cause or worsen a liver dysfunction [19-21].
- The increased risk of anastomotic leak due to splanchnic congestion if prolonged pedicle clamping is needed.
- The inadequate surgical exposure through a single incision.
- The need for a double surgical team for liver and colorectal surgery/inadequate treatment if a single team performs the entire procedure [21].
- The inability to select candidates for hepatic resection [22, 23].

Preliminary reports comparing simultaneous colorectal and liver surgery vs. delayed hepatectomies have noted increased morbidity and mortality rates in the first group [19, 20]. These data have not been confirmed by recent papers, in which similar short-term results between the two groups were described [9, 10, 14, 15, 17, 24, 25]. Furthermore, Martin et al., in assessing delayed liver resection data for both hospitalizations (colorectal resection and liver resection), reported a significantly lower morbidity rate and shorter hospital stay in patients who underwent simultaneous resection (49% vs. 67% and 12 vs. 18 days, respectively) [18]. The short-term results of delayed and simultaneous resections, reported by the most important surgical series, are summarized in Table 7.1.

After simultaneous colorectal and liver resection, two main complications are anticipated: anastomotic leak and liver dysfunction. The rate of anastomotic leak after simultaneous colorectal and liver resection is low and is similar to that of isolated colorectal resection [9, 10, 14, 15, 17, 18]. This result was achieved without enlarging the indications to diverting stoma. The risk of splanchnic congestion can be prevented by performing liver resection without pedicle clamping. If clamping is needed, intermittent occlusion may limit congestion and anastomosis can be performed after completion of the hepatectomy. Similarly, liver dysfunction rates were not increased in the simultaneous group.

Despite these encouraging data, the debate is still open and concerns which liver resections can be associated with colorectal surgery. The indications have been progressively enlarged [10, 17] and now include not only minor hepatectomies associated with right colectomies but, more recently, left colon-rectal surgery and major liver resections. Nonetheless, favorable data are based on series that mainly included minor resections; thus, many doubts persist if a major hepatectomy is planned. Recent papers reported high mortality rates after major liver surgery simultaneous to colorectal surgery: 25% in the series of Bolton et al. (2000) and in the series of Thelen et al. (2007) [26, 27]. These data were recently confirmed by a US multicenter database (MD Anderson Cancer Center, Houston; Johns Hopkins Medical Institutions, Baltimore; Duke University, Durham): mortality and morbidity were significantly higher in patients undergoing simultaneous major hepatectomy than in those in whom hepatectomy was delayed (8% vs. 1.4% and 44% vs. 27%, respectively) [28]. Our center recently published different results [17]:

Table 7.1 Short-term results after simultaneous colorectal and liver resection vs. delayed liver resection in patients with synchronous colorectal liver metastases

Author	Year	N S vs. D	Mortality			Morbidity		
			S	D	p^a	S	D	p^a
Nordlinger [20]	1996	115 vs. 893[b]	7%	2%	**0.005**			
Bolton [26]	2000	50 vs. 115[b]	12%	4%	n.s.			
Lyass [13]	2001	26 vs. 86	0%	2.3%	n.s.	27%	35%	n.s.
Weber [10]	2003	35 vs. 62	0%	0%	n.s.	23%	32%	n.s.
Martin [18][c]	2003	134 vs. 106	2%	2%	n.s.	49%	67%	**0.03**
Chua [14]	2004	64 vs. 32	0%	0%	n.s	53%	41%	n.s.
Tanaka [15]	2004	39 vs. 37	0%	0%	n.s	28%	16%	n.s
Thelen [27]	2007	40 vs. 179	10%	1.1%	**0.01**	18%	25%	n.s
Reddy [28]	2007	135 vs. 475	1%	0.5%	n.s.	36%	39%	n.s.
Martin [25]	2009	70 vs. 160	2%	2%	n.s.	56%	55%	n.s.
Brouquet [29]	2010	43 vs. 72	5%	3%	n.s.	47%	51%	n.s.
de Santibanes [24]	2010	185	1%			20.5%		
Capussotti[d]	2010	176 vs. 181	2%	1%	n.s.	33.0%	29.3%	n.s.
Major hepatectomies								
Bolton [26]	2000	17 vs. 27	23.5%	0%	**0.02**	-	-	-
Martin [18][c]	2003	45 vs. 76	4%	4%	n.s.	60%	70%	**0.03**
Thelen [27]	2007	15 vs. 142	26.7%	1.4%	**0.0007**	-	-	-
Reddy [28]	2007	36 vs. 291	8.3%	1.4%	**0.03**	44.4%	26.8%	**0.04**
Capussotti [17][c]	2007	31 vs. 48	3.2%	0%	*n.s.*	32.6%	56.3%	**0.04**
de Santibanes [24]	2010	42	4.7%			37.2%		

D, Delayed liver resection; *n.s.*, Not significant; *S,* Simultaneous colorectal and liver resection
[a]Significant values shown in bold
[b]Simultaneous colorectal and liver resection vs. other isolated liver resections
[c]In delayed liver resections, morbidity of both hospitalizations (colorectal surgery and liver surgery) is considered
[d] Unpublished data, updated to January 2010

31 consecutive patients who underwent major hepatectomy simultaneous with colorectal surgery had mortality and morbidity rates similar to those of 48 patients with delayed liver surgery (3% vs. 0% and 33% vs. 33%, respectively). Moreover, considering both hospitalizations in delayed procedures, overall hospital stay length, and morbidity rate were significantly lower after simultaneous resection (14 vs. 25 days and 33% vs. 56%, respectively). Martin et al. reported similar data in 2003 [18]. Interestingly, in the Berlin series of Thelen et al., all deaths occurred in elderly patients (over 70 years) [27]. De Santibanes et al. presented similar results: among 42 patients undergoing major liver resection simultaneous with colorectal resection, two deaths occurred (4.2%), both in patients older than 65 years [24]. Thus, a planned major liver resection should not be considered an absolute contraindication to simultaneous colorectal and liver resection, but extremely accurate patient selection is needed, especially in elderly patients.

A further problem of simultaneous resection may be the incision required to access such a large surgical field. Adequate surgical access can be guaranteed by an incision adapted to both the primary tumor and the liver metastases sites (Fig. 7.3): a right subcostal incision for right colon cancer, regardless of metastases localization; a midline incision for left colon-rectal cancer and left-sided metastases, associated with a right transverse supraumbilical incision if needed; a midline + right transverse supraumbilical incision or a double incision (midline + right subcostal) for left colon-rectal cancer and right-sided metastases [17] In some patients a midline incision is sufficient also for right-sided metastases.

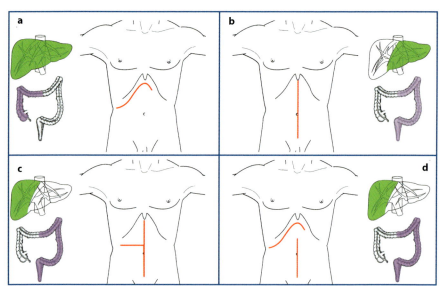

Fig. 7.3 Surgical incisions (*red line*) according to primary tumor (*violet area*) and liver metastases (*green area*) localizations. A right subcostal incision for right colon cancer, regardless of metastases localization (**a**); a midline incision for left colon cancer and left-sided metastases (**b**): a midline and right transverse supraumbilical incision (**c**) or a double incision, midline and right subcostal (**d**) for left colon-rectal cancer and right-sided metastases

The need for two different surgical teams specialized, respectively, in colorectal and hepatic surgery has never been confirmed. The achieved radicality rates and survival results suggest that simultaneous colorectal and liver resections can be safely performed in centers regularly treating both colorectal and hepatic neoplasms [8-10, 17].

Finally, some authors have suggested that delayed liver resection allows the evaluation of tumor biology and improved selection of good candidates for liver surgery [22, 23]. This issue needs to be clarified. As discussed below, immediate simultaneous colorectal and liver resection performed at diagnosis can be associated with a high risk of early and extensive recurrence because of microscopic neoplastic foci and unknown tumor biology. In these cases, a "time test" interval (see below) and/or neoadjuvant chemotherapy have been proposed. However, simultaneous resection is not synonymous with immediate resection at diagnosis. At present, neoadjuvant chemotherapy with the primary tumor still in situ can be performed, with subsequent planning of a simultaneous colorectal and liver resection. Furthermore, the hypothesized benefits from delayed liver resection in terms of patient selection have never been demonstrated: similar long-term results have been reported after simultaneous and delayed liver resections [8, 10, 13, 14, 29]. The results of the most important series are summarized in Table 7.2.

At present, the contraindications to simultaneous resection are [9, 10, 17, 18]:
1) emergency colorectal surgery;
2) low performance status/high ASA score;
3) impossibility to achieve radical resection.

Unexpected liver metastases detected at laparotomy for colorectal cancer do not represent an absolute contraindication to resection if complete thoraco-abdominal staging of the disease has been preoperatively performed and intraoperative ultrasonography is available to exclude further deposits.

Table 7.2 Survival results after simultaneous colorectal and liver resection vs. delayed liver resection in patients with synchronous colorectal liver metastases

Author	Year	N S vs. D	5-year survival		
			S	D	p
Fujita [16]	2000	83	31%		
Lyass[a] [13]	2001	26 vs. 86	28%	27%	n.s.
Weber [10]	2003	35 vs. 62	21%	22%	n.s.
Chua [14]	2004	64 vs. 32	28.9%	42.9%	n.s
Thelen [27]	2007	40 vs. 179	53%	39%	n.s.
Brouquet [29]	2010	43 vs. 72	55%	48%	n.s.
de Santibanes [24]	2010	185	36.1%		
Capussotti[b]	2010	176 vs. 181	37.2%	34.4%	n.s.

D, Delayed liver resection; S, Simultaneous colorectal and liver resection
[a]Synchronous vs. metachronous metastases
[b]Unpublished data updated to January 2010

In this debate, Mentha et al. advanced a novel "inverted" strategy in 2006 [30]. The authors planned a two-stage surgery in patients with synchronous liver metastases, with liver resection as the first procedure. The main advantage was the priority given to metastases treatment, as metastases are the true prognostic factor. A further advantage was the possibility to easily include radiation treatment before rectal surgery, whenever indicated. As discussed below, in the traditional treatment strategy the inclusion of radiotherapy represents a serious problem, and no definitive protocols have been established. Preliminary data on 20 patients were extremely good, with the reported survival rate 56% at 4 years. However, further studies are needed to validate this strategy.

7.2.2
Oncologic Issues

The management of patients with colorectal cancer and synchronous liver metastases has shifted towards a multidisciplinary strategy in which surgery plays a key role, but other treatments, such as chemotherapy and radiotherapy, have to be considered.

7.2.2.1
Time Test

In 2000, Makuuchi et al. suggested that the only contraindication to liver resection for colorectal liver metastases is the technical impossibility to achieve a complete resection [5]. This concept has been recently challenged by some oncologic considerations: among patients with technically resectable disease, neoadjuvant chemotherapy could help to distinguish between those who will truly benefit from surgery and those with rapidly progressive and thus incurable disease [22, 23]. The presence of liver metastases at diagnosis is an indicator of aggressive neoplastic disease. In resectable cases, up-front liver surgery has a double risk:

- It may be useless in patients with rapid and uncontrollable disease spread and progression.
- It may be inadequate because of possible microscopic neoplastic foci, which could lead to a high risk of early recurrence.

These considerations have led some authors to propose a time test, i.e., an interval of time before resection in order to better evaluate disease behavior and evolution [22, 23]. In 2000, Lambert et al. reported the first outcomes of this strategy [22]: 28 patients with resectable liver metastases synchronous to primary colorectal cancer were re-evaluated after a median observational interval of 5 months from diagnosis (during which only 13 patients received chemotherapy). In seven (25%) patients, new neoplastic foci were diagnosed and contraindicated resection. Compared with patients who underwent resection at diagnosis, the time test strategy did not worsen the whole-group results (mean survival 27 vs. 28 months), while it was associated with improved survival rates in the resected group (37 months). Yoshidome et al recently reported similar results [23]: among patients in whom liver resection was delayed after a time test interval, 43% developed additional metastatic lesions. After liver resection, the recurrence risk at 1 year was significantly lower in patients who had a time test before resection than in those who underwent resection at diagnosis (13% vs. 48%).

7.2.2.2
Neoadjuvant Chemotherapy

Preoperative chemotherapy administration is, theoretically, associated not only with time test advantages but also with tumor size reduction, enabling easier R0 resections, and the testing of the chemotherapy regimen in order to guide the choice of adjuvant treatments [31]. Unfortunately, few studies have addressed this issue.

In 2003, Allen et al. analyzed the long-term outcomes of 106 patients with synchronous liver metastases undergoing delayed liver resection and reported similar survival rates in patients with or without neoadjuvant chemotherapy [11]. However, the authors observed a significantly better survival in patients without progression while on neoadjuvant treatment than in untreated patients (5-year survival rate 87% vs. 38%). In 2008, a multicenter randomized controlled trial compared long-term outcomes of patients receiving chemotherapy before and after liver surgery with those of patients undergoing surgery alone [31]. The authors reported higher disease-free survival rates in treated patients. However, this study has been widely criticized, especially because the effects of pre- and postoperative chemotherapy cannot be distinguished. Finally, in 2009, a multi-institutional study collected data from 499 consecutive patients undergoing resection for synchronous colorectal liver metastases and specifically analyzed the impact of chemotherapy on their outcomes [32]. Postoperative, but not preoperative chemotherapy improved overall and disease-free survival. At present, the indications for neoadjuvant chemotherapy remain controversial.

In some centers, neoadjuvant chemotherapy is systematically administered to all patients with synchronous metastases. In others, there are attempts to identify the subgroups of patients who may benefit from preoperative treatment. In 2006, Minagawa et al. reported poor survival outcomes in patients with more than three lymph node metastases (median survival 1.8 vs. 3.3 years in the other patients) [12]. The authors proposed preoperative chemotherapy in these patients to better select candidates for resection, but this parameter is difficult to assess preoperatively. In 2006, our group analyzed a series of 127 consecutive patients undergoing surgery for synchronous metastases [8] and compared the outcomes of patients with and without time test (including preoperative chemotherapy). Two prognostic factors were identified: T4 stage of the primary tumor and number of liver metastases > 3. Patients with these negative prognostic factors had better survival rates if resection was performed after a time test period (60% vs. 17% and 34% vs. 15%, respectively). Following these results, in our center patients with > 3 metastases and/or suspected T4 primary colorectal cancer are regularly scheduled for neoadjuvant chemotherapy.

7.2.2.3
Neoadjuvant Radiotherapy/Radiochemotherapy

If liver resection is potentially a curative treatment in patients with synchronous liver metastases, it is necessary to plan the optimal treatment for the primary tumor, too. In case of mid/low rectal cancers, randomized controlled trials demonstrated a significant reduction of local relapse after neoadjuvant radiotherapy/radiochemotherapy [33, 34]. Theoretically, radiation should be included also in the treatment of patients with resectable synchronous metastases. A retrospective study from our group, in cooperation with the Cherqui group (Henri Mondor Hospital, Créteil, France), confirmed this hypothesis: among 50 patients with T3-T4 and/or N+ mid/low rectal tumor and synchronous liver metastases undergoing radical resection, the local recurrence rate was 15.6% in patients not receiving radiotherapy (unpublished data). This relapse rate is similar to that of non-metastatic patients. Furthermore, pelvic recurrences had a significant impact on prognosis.

In addition, the inclusion of radiotherapy in the treatment of patients with synchronous liver metastases presents some problems. Prognosis is related more to the metastases than to the primary tumor and high-dose systemic chemotherapy regimens are needed. However, if radiotherapy is included, chemotherapy doses have to be reduced [35]. Even if a chemotherapy effect on the primary tumor has been established [36], at present there are no data demonstrating its equivalence with radiation treatment.

The "inverted strategy" proposed by Mentha et al. (a two-step strategy in which liver resection is the first step and colorectal surgery the second) could offer a solution [30]: after complete removal of the liver disease, radiochemotherapy before rectal resection could be easily planned. Further strategies are possible, such as the inclusion of radiation in the last part of neoadjuvant treatment whenever resection is to be performed. Studies specifically focused on these options are needed to identify the optimal treatment strategy in these patients.

7.3
Unresectable Synchronous Liver Metastases

Synchronous liver metastases are unresectable in about 80–90% of patients, because of intrahepatic disease involvement or simultaneous extrahepatic metastases [1, 2] (Fig. 7.4). In these cases, chemotherapy is the ideal treatment, in order to improve the quality of life, prolong survival and, in some cases, to downsize the tumor thereby converting the patient disease to resectability (10–15%) [37, 38] (Fig. 7.5). The treatment strategy has to be modified according to the symptoms of the primary tumor.

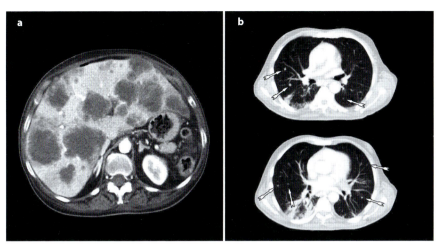

Fig. 7.4 Liver metastases synchronous to primary colorectal cancer that are unresectable because of massive liver involvement (**a**) or because of associated simultaneous multiple bilateral pulmonary metastases (**b**). *Arrows* indicate pulmonary metastases

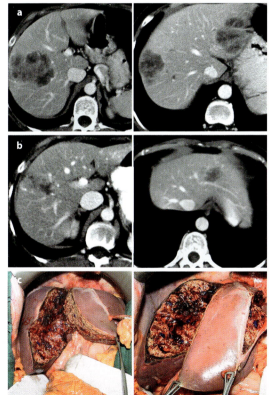

Fig. 7.5 Patient with initially unresectable metastases synchronous to primary sigmoid cancer undergoing liver resection after conversion chemotherapy. **a** CT scan at diagnosis; **b** CT after conversion chemotherapy; **c** surgical field after liver resection

7.3.1
Symptomatic Primary Tumor

In patients with symptomatic primary tumors (bleeding, occlusion, perforation), chemotherapy cannot be started and symptom treatment is required. If perforation of the primary tumor occurs, no solutions rather than surgery are available.

In case of occlusion, treatment is debated. Colorectal resection is commonly considered the gold standard treatment: it removes the obstruction, thus solving the occlusion, and allows complete disease staging, especially the disclosure of peritoneal carcinomatosis [39-41]. Unfortunately, resection is associated with high mortality and morbidity rates (up to 10% and 48%, respectively). Furthermore, access to chemotherapy is delayed. A diverting stoma without resection could represent an alternative because of lower morbidity rates and shorter postoperative recovery, but symptom relief is less effective [40].

Recently, endoscopic metallic stents have been proposed [42-44] (Fig. 7.6). Retrospective series have compared the outcomes of endoscopic stent and colorectal resection in these patients. Endoscopic stents were associated with lower morbidity rates, a reduced need for diverting stoma, shorter hospitalization, and faster access to chemotherapy [42-44]. In addition, endoscopic treatment may allow the completion of preoperative staging in patients with occlusive cancer at diagnosis, in order to choose the optimal treatment strategy. In 2007, Karoui et al. demonstrated that even tumors in the transverse and the right colon could be treated by endoscopic stents [44]. At present, contraindications to this procedure are primary tumor of the mid-low rectum because of stent-related symptoms, suspected ischemic lesions of the cecum secondary to colonic distension, and multiple colonic obstructions and/or associated ileal stenosis (i.e., peritoneal carcinomatosis) [44]. Stent placement can be associated with some complications, the most important being tumor perforation, which has been reported in about 5–10% of patients. Other adverse events include stent displacement or obstruction, but in both cases an endoscopic solution can be

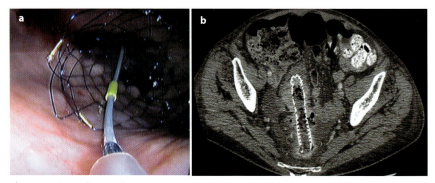

Fig. 7.6 Endoscopic metallic stent for obstructive primary colorectal tumor. **a** Endoscopic view while positioning; **b** CT scan after endoscopic metallic stent positioning

attempted. The effect of endoscopic stenting on prognosis is not yet clear, even if preliminary data have reported similar survival rates after stent positioning and resection. Larger prospective analysis and randomized trials are needed to validate this procedure in terms of effectiveness and safety. Furthermore, few centers systematically consider endoscopic treatment for patients with occlusive metastatic tumor because of different endoscopy expertise and organizational problems.

In case of mid-low rectal tumor, local excision or radiation treatments may be effective in symptom control but these procedures are beyond the scope of this chapter.

7.3.2
Asymptomatic Primary Tumor

Even in patients with asymptomatic primary tumor, colorectal surgery has traditionally represented the up-front treatment before chemotherapy. The priority given to colorectal surgery was justified by the fear of intestinal occlusion in patients on chemotherapy, thus requiring high-risk emergency surgery. Recent multicenter surveys confirm that this is still the more commonly adopted strategy [45,46]: up to 75% of patients in UK and US hospitals receive colorectal resection even for asymptomatic stage IV diseases. However, epidemiological data and recent chemotherapy progresses have challenged this attitude for the following reasons:
- Prognosis is determined by distant metastases more than by primary colorectal cancer.
- In the natural history of stage IV colorectal cancer, asymptomatic patients do not develop primary tumor-related symptoms in a high proportion of cases.
- Chemotherapy administration is the priority and is associated with prolonged survival;
- Chemotherapy is effective not only on metastatic sites, but also on the primary tumor (Fig. 7.7).

Based on these data, a new therapeutic strategy has been proposed: up-front chemotherapy with primary tumor in place [47-53]. The results of series in which this strategy was employed are summarized in Table 7.3. Except for the series by Ruo et al. of 2003, in which emergency surgery while on chemotherapy was required in 30% of the patients [54], low occlusion risk (9–20%) was reported [47, 49-53]. The survival rates of patients with up-front chemotherapy and of those receiving immediate surgery were similar [47, 49-53]. In 2005, Benoist at al. published a case-control study comparing results of the two strategies [49]: 27 patients with asymptomatic colorectal cancer and unresectable synchronous liver metastases receiving up-front chemotherapy without initial primary resection were compared with 32 patients treated initially by resection of the primary tumor. The chemotherapy group had more rapid access to chemotherapy (mean delay 15 vs. 44 days), shorter hospitalization length (mean 11 vs. 22 days), and similar survival (median 23 vs. 22 months). Palliative surgery was needed in 15% of the patients. In 2007, our group reported a prospective series of 35 patients with stage IV unresectable colorectal cancer who underwent up-front chemotherapy with the primary tumor in place [47]. All patients

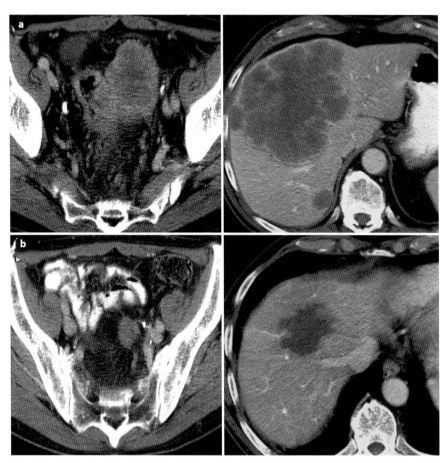

Fig. 7.7 Response of both primary tumor and synchronous liver metastases to chemotherapy. **a** CT scan at diagnosis; **b** CT after chemotherapy

received oxaliplatin-based chemotherapy, while in previous series isolated 5-FU was administered to a large number of patients. In our study, the disease became secondarily resectable in 13 patients (37.1%). Only one patient (2.8%) required emergency surgery and a diverting stoma because of intestinal occlusion. These results were recently confirmed by a large series including 233 patients, all treated by up-front oxaliplatin and/or irinotecan chemotherapy [53]: palliative surgery was required in 7% of the patients and radical resection was possible in 20%. The effectiveness of chemotherapy probably had a key-role in reducing occlusion risk. In fact, a similar regression grade in primary tumor and liver metastases was recently reported [36]. A cautionary note is needed about bevacizumab administration in patients with primary tumor in place because intestinal perforations have been reported.

Table 7.3 Results of up-front chemotherapy with primary tumor in place in patients with unresectable stage IV colorectal cancer

Author	Year	N	Chemotherapy	Follow-up (months)	Palliative surgery[a]	Curative surgery[b]
Scoggins [48]	1999	23	5-FU	-	2 (8.7%)	0
Sarela [52]	2001	24	5-FU[c]	18	4 (16.7%)	1 (4.2%)
Ruo [54]	2003	103	5-FU	-	30 (29%)	0
Tebutt [50]	2003	82	5-FU	19	8 (9.8%)	0
Michel [51]	2004	23	Oxaliplatin/Irinotecan[d]	19	5 (21.7%)	2 (8.7%)
Benoist [49]	2005	27	Oxaliplatin/Irinotecan[e]	22	4 (14.8%)	6 (22.2%)
Muratore [47]	2007	35	Oxaliplatin	26	1 (2.8%)	13 (37.1%)
Poultsides [53]	2009	233	Oxaliplatin/Irinotecan	NR	16 (7%)	47 (20%)

5-FU, 5-Fluorouracil; NR, data not reported
[a]Patients who needed surgery for primary tumor complications
[b]Patients in whom tumor resection was performed secondary to downsizing
[c]No chemotherapy: 4 patients; de Gramont regimen: 14 patients; oxaliplatin or irinotecan: 6 patients
[d]Oxaliplatin: 80% of patients
[e]Oxaliplatin or Irinotecan: 18 patients

A further point in favour of up-front chemotherapy is the availability of stents in case of occlusion during treatment. Successful endoscopic stent positioning avoids laparotomy and may allow chemotherapy to be continued. In 2010, Karoui et al. reported a prospective series of 68 patients with unresectable stage IV colorectal cancer [55]: 37 received up-front chemotherapy, with stent insertion in 19. Among them, nine had intestinal occlusion while on chemotherapy, which was solved by stent placement in two third of cases. In the whole series of 68 patients, median survival was 6.4 months, but it reached 15.4 months considering the up-front chemotherapy group ($p < 0.0001$). These data further suggest the fundamental role of a multidisciplinary approach to these patients to optimize treatment strategy and improve outcomes.

7.4
Conclusions

Radical surgery is the gold standard in the treatment of synchronous colorectal liver metastases. It prolongs patient survival and is potentially curative in some cases.

Simultaneous colorectal and liver resection can be safely performed if minor hepatectomies are needed. The results are similar to those obtained with a delayed procedure, and even better in some studies. If a major hepatectomy is required, the results of simultaneous colorectal and liver resection are controversial.

Neoadjuvant chemotherapy helps to better select candidates for surgery, but at present there is no evidence in favour of its systematic application. Selected patients may benefit from neoadjuvant chemotherapy, such as those with more than three metastases. It can be performed with the primary tumor in place, planning a simultaneous colorectal and hepatic resection at the end of treatment.

In patients with unresectable synchronous liver metastases, chemotherapy is the treatment of choice. In asymptomatic patients, chemotherapy should be immediately started with the primary tumor in place. The risk of occlusion is low, especially if modern chemotherapy regimens are administered. In patients with a symptomatic primary tumor, chemotherapy has to be preceded by symptoms treatment. Endoscopic metallic stents may represent an effective alternative to surgery in the treatment of occlusive symptoms.

Clearly, a multidisciplinary approach is mandatory in patients with primary colorectal cancer and synchronous liver metastases, in order to define the optimal treatment strategy which must be tailored to every single patient.

References

1. Manfredi S, Lepage C, Hatem C et al (2006) Epidemiology and management of liver metastases from colorectal cancer. Ann Surg 244:254-259
2. Simmonds PC, Primrose JN, Colquitt JL et al (2006) Surgical resection of hepatic metastases from colorectal cancer: a systematic review of published studies. Br J Cancer 94:982-999
3. Wagner JS, Adson MA, Van Heerden JA et al (1984) The natural history of hepatic metastases from colorectal cancer. A comparison with resective treatment. Ann Surg 199:502-508
4. Scheele J, Stangl R, Altendorf-Hofmann A (1990) Hepatic metastases from colorectal carcinoma: impact of surgical resection on the natural history. Br J Surg 77:1241-1246
5. Minagawa M, Makuuchi M, Torzilli G et al (2000) Extension of the frontiers of surgical indications in the treatment of liver metastases from colorectal cancer: long-term results. Ann Surg 231:487-499
6. Tomlinson JS, Jarnagin WR, DeMatteo RP et al (2007) Actual 10-year survival after resection of colorectal liver metastases defines cure. J Clin Oncol 25:4575-4580
7. Viganò L, Ferrero A, Lo Tesoriere R et al (2008) Liver surgery for colorectal metastases: results after 10 years of follow-up. Long-term survivors, late recurrences, and prognostic role of morbidity. Ann Surg Oncol 15:2458-2464
8. Capussotti L, Viganò L, Ferrero A et al (2007) Timing of resection of liver metastases synchronous to colorectal tumor: proposal of prognosis-based decisional model. Ann Surg Oncol 14:1143-1150
9. de Santibanes E, Lassalle FB, McCormack L et al (2002) Simultaneous colorectal and hepatic resections for colorectal cancer: postoperative and longterm outcomes. J Am Coll Surg 195:196–202
10. Weber JC, Bachellier P, Oussoultzoglou E et al (2003) Simultaneous resection of colorectal primary tumor and synchronous liver metastases. Br J Surg 90:956–962
11. Allen PJ, Kemeny N, Jarnagin W et al (2003) Importance of response to neoadjuvant chemotherapy in patients undergoing resection of synchronous colorectal liver metastases. J Gastroin-

7 Synchronous Colorectal Liver Metastases

test Surg 7:109-115

12. Minagawa M, Yamamoto J, Miwa S et al (2006) Selection criteria for simultaneous resection in patients with synchronous liver metastasis. Arch Surg 141:1006-1012
13. Lyass S, Zamir G, Matot I et al (2001) Combined colon and hepatic resection for synchronous colorectal liver metastases. J Surg Oncol 78:17–21
14. Chua HK, Sondenaa K, Tsiotos GG et al (2004) Concurrent vs staged colectomy and hepatectomy for primary colorectal cancer with synchronous hepatic metastases. Dis Colon Rectum 47:1310–1316
15. Tanaka K, Shimada H, Matsuo K et al (2004) Outcome after simultaneous colorectal and hepatic resection for colorectal cancer with synchronous metastases. Surgery 136:650–659
16. Fujita S, Akasu T, Moriya Y (2000) Resection of synchronous liver metastases from colorectal cancer. Jpn J Clin Oncol 30:7–11
17. Capussotti L, Ferrero A, Viganò L et al (2007) Major liver resections synchronous with colorectal surgery. Ann Surg Oncol 14:195-201
18. Martin R, Paty P, Fong Y et al (2003) Simultaneous liver and colorectal resections are safe for synchronous colorectal liver metastasis. J Am Coll Surg 197:233–241
19. Vogt P, Raab R, Ringe B et al (1991) Resection of synchronous liver metastases from colorectal cancer. World J Surg 15:62–67
20. Nordlinger B, Guiguet M, Vaillant JC et al (1996) Surgical resection of colorectal carcinoma metastases to the liver. A prognostic scoring system to improve case selection, based on 1568 patients. Association Française de Chirurgie. Cancer 77:1254-1262
21. Belghiti J (1990) Synchronous and resectable hepatic metastases of colorectal cancer: should there be a minimum delay before hepatic resection? Ann Chir 44:427–429
22. Lambert LA, Colacchio TA, Barth RJ Jr (2000) Interval hepatic resection of colorectal metastases improves patient selection. Arch Surg 135:473-479
23. Yoshidome H, Kimura F, Shimizu H et al (2008) Interval period tumor progression: does delayed hepatectomy detect occult metastases in synchronous colorectal liver metastases? J Gastrointest Surg 12:1391-1398
24. de Santibañes E, Fernandez D, Vaccaro C et al (2010) Short-Term and Long-Term Outcomes After Simultaneous Resection of Colorectal Malignancies and Synchronous Liver Metastases. World J Surg in press
25. Martin RC 2nd, Augenstein V, Reuter NP et al (2009) Simultaneous versus staged resection for synchronous colorectal cancer liver metastases. J Am Coll Surg 208:842-850
26. Bolton JS, Fuhrman GM (2000) Survival after resection of multiple bilobar hepatic metastases from colorectal carcinoma. Ann Surg 231:743–751
27. Thelen A, Jonas S, Benckert C et al (2007) Simultaneous versus staged liver resection of synchronous liver metastases from colorectal cancer. Int J Colorectal Dis 22:1269-1276
28. Reddy SK, Pawlik TM, Zorzi D et al (2007) Simultaneous resections of colorectal cancer and synchronous liver metastases: a multi-institutional analysis. Ann Surg Oncol 14:3481-3491
29. Brouquet A, Mortenson MM, Vauthey JN et al (2010) Surgical strategies for synchronous colorectal liver metastases in 156 consecutive patients: classic, combined or reverse strategy? J Am Coll Surg 210:934-941
30. Mentha G, Majno PE, Andres A et al (2006) Neoadjuvant chemotherapy and resection of advanced synchronous liver metastases before treatment of the colorectal primary. Br J Surg 93:872-878
31. Nordlinger B, Sorbye H, Glimelius B et al (2008) Perioperative chemotherapy with FOLFOX4 and surgery versus surgery alone for resectable liver metastases from colorectal cancer: a randomised controlled trial. Lancet 371:1007-1016
32. Reddy SK, Zorzi D, Lum YW et al (2009) Timing of multimodality therapy for resectable synchronous colorectal liver metastases: a retrospective multi-institutional analysis. Ann Surg Oncol 16:1809-1819

33. Kapiteijn E, Marijnen CA, Nagtegaal ID et al (2001) Preoperative radiotherapy combined with total mesorectal excision for resectable rectal cancer. N Engl J Med 345:638–646

34. Bosset JF, Collette L, Calais G et al (2006) Chemotherapy with preoperative radiotherapy in rectal cancer. N Engl J Med 355:1114–1123

35. Benoist S (2007) Recommendations for clinical practice. Therapeutic choices for rectal cancer. How should rectal cancers with synchronous metastases be managed? Gastroenterol Clin Biol 31:1S75-80S100-102

36. Karoui M, Koubaa W, Delbaldo C et al (2008) Chemotherapy has also an effect on primary tumor in colon carcinoma. Ann Surg Oncol 15:3440-3446

37. Adam R, Delvart V, Pascal G et al (2004) Rescue surgery for unresectable colorectal liver metastases downstaged by chemotherapy: a model to predict long-term survival. Ann Surg 240:644-657

38. Capussotti L, Muratore A, Mulas MM et al (2006) Neoadjuvant chemotherapy and resection for initially irresectable colorectal liver metastases. Br J Surg 93:1001-1006

39. Joffe J, Gordon PH (1981) Palliative resection for colorectal carcinoma. Dis Colon rectum 24:355–360

40. Longo WE, Ballantyne GH, Bilchik AJ et al (1988) Advanced rectal cancer. What is the best palliation? Dis Colon Rectum 31:842–847

41. Nash GM, Saltz LB, Kemeny NE et al (2002) Radical resection of rectal cancer primary tumor provides effective local therapy in patients with stage IV disease. Ann Surg Oncol 9:954-960

42. Law WL, Choi HK, Chu KW (2003) Comparison of stenting with emergency surgery as palliative treatment for obstructing primary left-sided colorectal cancer. Br J Surg 90:1429-1433

43. Carne PW, Frye JN, Robertson GM et al (2004) Stents or open operation for palliation of colorectal cancer: a retrospective, cohort study of perioperative outcome and long-term survival. Dis Colon Rectum 47:1455-1461

44. Karoui M, Charachon A, Delbaldo C et al (2007) Stents for palliation of obstructive metastatic colon cancer: impact on management and chemotherapy administration. Arch Surg 142:619-623

45. Mella J, Biffin A, Radcliffe AG et al (1997) Population-based audit of colorectal cancer management in two UK health regions. Colorectal Cancer Working Group, Royal College of Surgeons of England Clinical Epidemiology and Audit Unit. Br J Surg 84:1731-1736

46. Temple LK, Hsieh L, Wong WD et al (2004) Use of surgery among elderly patients with stage IV colorectal cancer. J Clin Oncol 22:3475-3484

47. Muratore A, Zorzi D, Bouzari H et al (2007) Asymptomatic colorectal cancer with un-resectable liver metastases: immediate colorectal resection or up-front systemic chemotherapy? Ann Surg Oncol 14:766-770

48. Scoggins CR, Meszoely IM, Blanke CD et al (1999) Nonoperative management of primary colorectal cancer in patients with stage IV disease. Ann Surg Oncol 6:651–657

49. Benoist S, Pautrat K, Mitry E et al (2005) Treatment strategy for patients with colorectal cancer and synchronous irresectable liver metastases. Br J Surg 92:1155–1160

50. Tebbutt NC, Norman AR, Cunningham D et al (2003) Intestinal complications after chemotherapy for patients with unresected primary colorectal cancer and synchronous metastases. Gut 52:568–573

51. Michel P, Roque I, Di Fiore F et al (2004) Colorectal cancer with non-resectable synchronous metastases: should the primary tumor be resected? Gastroenterol Clin Biol 28:434–437

52. Sarela AI, Guthrie JA, Seymour MT et al (2001) Non-operative management of the primary tumor in patients with incurable stage IV colorectal cancer. Br J Surg 88:1352-1356

53. Poultsides GA, Servais EL, Saltz LB et al (2009) Outcome of primary tumor in patients with synchronous stage IV colorectal cancer receiving combination chemotherapy without surgery as initial treatment. J Clin Oncol 27:3379-3384

54. Ruo L, Gougoutas C, Paty PB et al (2003) Elective bowel resection for incurable stage IV colorectal cancer: prognostic variables for asymptomatic patients. J Am Coll Surg 196:722–728
55. Karoui M, Soprani A, Charachon A et al (2010) Primary chemotherapy with or without colonic stent for management of irresectable stage IV colorectal cancer. Eur J Surg Oncol 36:58-64

Therapeutic Strategies in Unresectable Colorectal Liver Metastases

8

Abstract The majority of patients with colorectal liver metastases presents with unresectable disease at diagnosis, because of the size, location, or extent of the tumor. While chemotherapy remains the first option for these patients, only multimodal management can increase the resectability rates. When patients cannot be safely operated on because the future liver remnant after the scheduled hepatectomy would be too small, portal vein occlusion is a safe procedure to decrease the risk of postoperative liver failure. Two-stage hepatectomy and associated interstitial treatments are effective strategies in case of multiple bilateral metastases.

8.1
Introduction

Radical surgical resection is the only potentially curative treatment modality for patients with colorectal liver metastases. Nevertheless, in the majority of patients the liver is deemed to be unresectable at diagnosis, because of the size, location, or extent of disease. In these particular cases, management should be multimodal, with the collaboration of surgeons, oncologists, radiologists, and gastroenterologists. Chemotherapy remains the first option for patients with initially unresectable disease and its role has been previously discussed in this volume. Sometimes patients cannot be safely operated on because the future liver remnant after the scheduled hepatectomy would be too small. In such cases, portal vein occlusion has been introduced to decrease the risk of postoperative liver failure. Two-stage hepatectomy strategy and associated interstitial treatments are effective procedures in patients with multiple bilateral metastases

A. Ferrero (✉)
Division of Hepato-Bilio-Pancreatic and Digestive Surgery, Mauriziano "Umberto I" Hospital, Turin, Italy

Surgical Treatment of Colorectal Liver Metastases. Lorenzo Capussotti (Ed.)
© Springer-Verlag Italia 2011

8.2
Portal Vein Occlusion

The onset of postoperative liver failure is still a serious complication after major liver resection. Patients with colorectal liver metastases who undergo preoperative chemotherapy are at particular risk. To prevent post-hepatectomy liver insufficiency, preoperative portal vein embolization (PVE) can be performed. This procedure was first introduced into clinical practice for patients with hilar cholangiocarcinoma. The rationale is to occlude a branch of the portal venous flow, which subsequently leads to ipsilateral hepatic atrophy and compensatory contralateral hypertrophy. A second advantage is the reduction of post-hepatectomy portal pressure; this is particularly useful in patients with liver cirrhosis and in patients scheduled for simultaneous liver and colorectal resections with intestinal anastomosis.

8.2.1
Indications

There is a general consensus that patients with a future liver remnant (FLR) < 25% of the total functioning hepatic volume have an increased risk of postoperative liver dysfunction and should undergo preoperative portal vein occlusion [1]. Nevertheless, some authors have reported series of patients undergoing PVE that included patients with a calculated FLR > 25%. In the series of Imamura et al., 84 patients underwent PVE before extensive liver surgery [2]; their indications for this procedure included a planned hepatectomy corresponding to the removal of > 55% of the total hepatic parenchyma, independent of both the indications for surgery and liver function. Azoulay et al. suggested that, when liver function is impaired by neoadjuvant chemotherapy, postoperative complications can be reduced by ensuring that at least 40% of total hepatic volume remains [3]. We recently reported the results of a prospective study correlating FLR with early surgical outcomes. The goal of that study was to identify the critical residual volume associated with postoperative hepatic dysfunction. This was determined to be 26.5% in patients with normal liver function and 31% in patients with suspected preoperative impaired liver function [4].

8.2.2
Techniques of Portal Vein Occlusion

Both PVE and portal vein ligature (PVL) are good options to occlude a branch of the portal vein. Two different methods have been reported to access the portal vein for embolization: transileocolic portal embolization and percutaneous transhepatic portal embolization. In the first procedure, a mini-laparotomy is performed, with the patient under general anesthesia to facilitate insertion of the catheter into the portal vein through a branch of the ileocolic vein. A diagnostic laparoscopy and laparoscopic ultrasound scan can be performed during the procedure, providing further accurate staging of the disease. Percutaneous access to the portal venous system is safe and relatively simple and can be performed with the patient under local anesthesia. The approach may be transhepatic ipsilateral or contralateral. The ipsilateral approach (Fig. 8.1) is technically more demanding but has the advantage that, since the FLR is not instrumented, the risk of portal vein thrombosis and vascular injury is minimized. Many available embolic agents, such as polyvinyl alcohol, microcoil, gelfoam, and cyanoacrylate, have been used for preoperative PVE, without significant differences in degrees or rates of hypertrophy of the non-embolized segments. Complications are infrequent after PVE, the most common post-procedural findings being fever and abdominal discomfort or pain. Di Stefano et al. reported the occurrence of adverse events in 24 (12.8%) of 188 patients, including 12 complications and 12 incidental imaging findings [5].

Portal vein occlusion is easily done by surgical ligature (PVL) when a laparotomy is requested to resect the colon primary tumor or to remove metastases in the left liver in a two-stage strategy. PVE was initially reported to produce a significantly greater increase in remnant liver volume and shorter hospital stay than PVL [6]. However, we recently reported a study comparing 17 patients who underwent PVL with 31 patients treated by preoperative PVE. PVL was demonstrated to be safe, providing similar rates of hypertrophy as PVE [7].

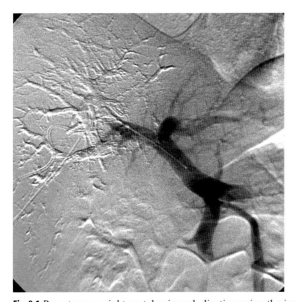

Fig. 8.1 Percutaneous right portal vein embolization using the ipsilateral approach

8.2.3
Future Liver Remnant Hypertrophy After PVE

Post-embolization imaging is essential for the assessment of changes in liver volume and the planning of liver resection. A volumetric study is usually performed by CT scan or MRI. The average interval for the volumetric study from portal vein occlusion to surgery is 3–4 weeks. The calculated range of percentage increase of FLR volume following PVE was 8–27% in a recent meta-analysis covering 37 publications [8]. Routine embolization of Sg4 portal branches combined with right PVE has been suggested in patients who are candidates for right trisectionectomy, to induce greater and faster hypertrophy of the remnant liver. This approach may, however, increase the risk of accidental occlusion of the left portal branches, thus precluding surgery. We demonstrated that the rates of volume increase were similar in patients who underwent right PVE with or without embolization of the Sg4 portal branches [9]. The degree of hypertrophy, together with the FLR volume, was reported to be a significant predictor of postoperative hepatic dysfunction [10].

Clinical and experimental data suggest that tumor progression can occur after preoperative PVE in embolized and non-embolized liver segments. Three possible mechanisms influencing tumor growth after PVE can be recognized, namely, changes in cytokines or growth factors, alterations in hepatic blood supply, and an enhanced cellular host response promoting local tumor growth after PVE [11]. Elias was the first to point out the risk after PVE or PVL of inducing rapid growth of potential tumors in the hypertrophic left lateral segments and of the tumor to be resected [12]. These findings were confirmed by Kokudo et al., who demonstrated a tumor volume increase after PVE, both in embolized and non-embolized parenchyma. Tumor growth was determined based on the Ki-67 labeling index of metastatic lesions, which was higher in patients who had undergone PVE [13]. These data suggest that metastases within the FLR should be treated before scheduling PVE.

8.2.4
Chemotherapy and Hypertrophy

Patients with advanced metastatic disease are usually referred for surgery when neoadjuvant chemotherapy has been performed. It is commonly believed that chemotherapy impairs FLR hypertrophy after PVE. The rationale for this comes from experimental models in which an ability of antimitotic agents to interfere with liver-resection-induced regeneration was demonstrated [14]. Goere et al. compared ten patients in whom oxaliplatin- or irinotecan based chemotherapy was maintained until surgery after portal vein occlusion with ten patients in whom chemotherapy was interrupted at least one month prior to portal obstruction. The FLR increase was comparable in the two groups [15]. The use of bevacizumab, a monoclonal antibody that targets vascular endothelial growth factor (VEGF) and inhibits the angiogenesis, could theoretically impair the parenchymal response to PVE. Zorzi et al. reported no differences in the degree of FLR hypertrophy after PVE among patients treated with

8 Therapeutic Strategies in Unresectable Colorectal Liver Metastases   125

or without preoperative chemotherapy with bevacizumab [16]. Nevertheless, in both groups, chemotherapy was suspended 7 weeks before PVE. In a recent paper, Aussilhou et al. reported a smaller increase in FLR in patients previously treated with bevacizumab, particularly if they underwent six or more cycles and were older than 60 years [17]. We actually recommend stopping bevacizumab earlier than other chemotherapy agents and to avoid its use between portal occlusion and surgery.

8.2.5
Early Outcomes of Hepatectomies Following PVE

Before surgery, imaging re-evaluation is mandatory not only to assess FLR hypertrophy but also to investigate tumor progression. Following PVE, about 68% of patients undergo their scheduled major hepatectomy. Patients are excluded from surgery before or during laparotomy on the basis of inadequate FLR hypertrophy, progression of liver metastases, or development of pulmonary metastases or extrahepatic spread.

Hemming et al. compared 31 patients who underwent extended hepatectomy after PVE to 21 patients with similar characteristics who had an extended hepatectomy without PVE [18]. Mortality rates were similar, but postoperative peak bilirubin was higher in the non-PVE than in the PVE group, as were postoperative fresh-frozen plasma requirements. Transient liver failure (33% vs. 10%, $p = 0.03$) and hospital stay, by contrast, were higher in the non-PVE patients. A recent meta-analysis including 1088 patients who underwent PVE reported overall morbidity and mortality rates following hepatectomy of 16% and 1.7%, respectively [8]. Transient liver failure was rarely observed (2.5% of cases) but seven patients developed acute liver failure and died (0.8%). Other causes of death were portal vein thrombosis (3 patients) and sepsis. Even in the absence of a randomized trial to confirm this conclusion, it seems that PVE decreases the risk of onset of postoperative liver failure.

8.2.6
Long-term Results

The survival of patients with initially unresectable colorectal liver metastases who underwent hepatectomy after PVE is considerably longer than that of patients who did not undergo hepatic resection. In the recently published Paul Brousse Hospital experience, overall 3-year survival was 44% and 0%, respectively [19]. Nevertheless, there is disagreement in the literature about the prognostic role of PVE in the long-term results of patients undergoing radical hepatectomy. In a recent study comparing 36 patients treated by right/extended right hepatectomy after PVE with 65 patients receiving the same operation but without PVE, the reported 5-year survival after liver resection was 25% with PVE and 50% without PVE [20]. Even disease-free survival was poorer for patients with PVE. The same results were reported by Kokudo et al.: while overall survival was similar in the two groups, patients with preoperative PVE had significantly lower disease-free survival rates than those in the non-PVE group

(15.2% vs 45.8% and 0% vs 34.4% at 2 and 4 years, respectively) [13]. However, PVE was reported to decrease intrahepatic recurrence rates (26.0% vs. 76.1% in patients without PVE), suggesting that preoperative PVE contributes to reducing intrahepatic tumoral spreading by intraluminal occlusion of the peripheral portal branches [21]. In conclusion, even if PVE is effective in extending the indications for surgery in patients with initially unresectable colorectal metastases, to date, patient selection for PVE should be done cautiously.

8.3
Two-stage Hepatectomy

Although hepatic resection is the treatment of choice for patients with colorectal liver metastases, on presentation, between 75% and 85% of these patients are not candidates for surgery. In particular, a substantial number of patients who present with extensive bilateral and multinodular metastatic liver disease are deemed to have unresectable disease by standard criteria. In fact, in the presence of intrahepatic multinodular tumor diffusion, curative resection is surgically impossible as all liver metastases cannot be completely removed while preserving an adequate FLR [22]. Yet, an incomplete resection is contraindicated because it has been demonstrated that there is no significant survival benefit compared with patients who do not undergo surgery [23].

8.3.1
Strategies

In patients in whom complete extirpation of the metastases by a single hepatectomy is not feasible, treatment consisting of sequential hepatectomies has been advocated by Adam et al. [24]. In their seminal proposal, the authors devised a surgical strategy, termed two-stage hepatectomy, whose overall intention is curative but in which the initial stage of the hepatic resection aimed at removing the highest possible number of metastases, but not all of them. The initial operation is then followed by a period of time to allow hypertrophy of the remaining liver. A second, curative-intent operation is then performed to resect the remaining disease, after adequate parenchymal hypertrophy has reduced the risk of postoperative liver insufficiency. Due to the lack of a standardized approach to this strategy, in 2004 Jaeck et al. [25] proposed a modified two-stage program to systematically include, after the first hepatic resection, PVE, which minimizes the risk of postoperative liver insufficiency. In the initial operation, low-volume disease is extirpated in the planned FLR, usually the left lobe, through wedge resections with or without local destructive techniques. Performing the minor hepatectomy first enables protection of the FLR by avoiding manipulation and resection in a small, friable, hypertrophic remnant, which would be required if the minor resection were performed second. In addition, repeat dissection of the remnant and associated adhesions at the time of planned second-stage major resection is avoided. Furthermore, if the disease progresses between stages, the patient is spared the morbidity of a major hepatectomy. Finally, resection first of the metastatic deposits in the FLR prevents the tumor overgrowth observed after PVE [12].

In patients with synchronous bilobar liver metastases and the primary tumor in place, the two-stage approach is particularly attractive because it allows the primary tumor to be treated during the first liver stage. This decreases the number of surgical procedures with repetitive imunosuppression from multiple major surgeries, avoids delay in adjuvant chemotherapy, and allows for a precise staging of metastatic disease during the colectomy. In addition, the first stage focuses on the "easy side" of the liver, with minor hepatic resection performed at the same time of colectomy, while major hepatectomy is left for a second specific stage (Fig. 8.2) [26-28]. As we recently showed in a bi-institutional study, this strategy prevents the occurrence of liver-specific complications at the time of colorectal resection which, per se, is a major procedure carrying risks for severe complications, such as anastomotic leak [28].

Patients selected for a two-stage procedure are at high risk of tumor progression during the period of liver hypertrophy. Thus, the use of chemotherapy during this interval has been proposed. Although its effectiveness with regard to survival, perioperative morbidity, and mortality has not yet been elucidated, data indicate that chemotherapy can be safely administered. Goere et al. [15] recently observed that the administration of oxaliplatin- or irinotecan-based chemotherapy after PVE did not

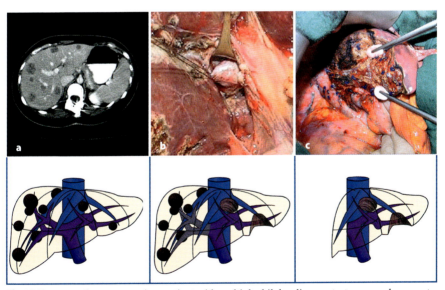

Fig. 8.2 Two-stage hepatectomy in a patient with multiple, bilobar liver metastases synchronous to a right colon adenocarcinoma. The volume of the left liver was 24% of the total liver volume. **a** Preoperative CT scan. **b** Clearance of the left hemi-liver at the time of the primary resection with concurrent right portal vein ligation. **c** Right hepatectomy performed 6 weeks later, after compensatory hypertrophy of the left liver (32% of the total liver volume)

impair liver hypertrophy compared to patients in whom chemotherapy was interrupted one month before PVE. This is consistent with the findings of others showing that preoperative chemotherapy does not affect postoperative liver regeneration [29]. However, the safety of bevacizumab during the waiting time between the two resections is controversial [16, 17]. Nevertheless, because of the potential to reduce the rate of liver hypertrophy, especially after prolonged pre-PVE chemotherapy, the use of bevacizumab is not recommended.

As previously discussed, ligation of the right portal vein has been demonstrated, in both the experimental and the clinical setting, to induce hypertrophy of the left liver to a similar magnitude as achieved with PVE [7]. Therefore, PVL may be an alternative to postoperative PVE. However, when the extent of resection in the FLR is substantial, it might be preferable to perform PVE 5–7 days after resection, to minimize the risk of postoperative hepatic insufficiency and to provide a further impulse to the already regenerating liver.

8.3.2
Short- and Long-term Results

Table 8.1 reports technical aspects, short- and long-term outcomes following two-stage hepatectomy in selected single and bi-institutional cohorts. In the first published series by Adam et al. [24] 16 patients were initially treated but only 13 (81%) actually underwent the second hepatectomy. Recently, the same authors updated their experience, showing that among 59 patients in whom a two-stage approach was initially planned only 69% successfully completed curative-intent treatment [30]. This rate is similar to that reported by others, which varies between 70% and 78% [25, 28, 31, 32]. In the vast majority of cases, patients failed to complete the second procedure because of tumor progression within or outside the liver. This observation points out the importance of chemotherapy responsiveness on the outcome of these patients and the need for a careful patient selection. Tsai et al. [32] observed that patients who did not complete the two-stage approach were more likely to have received preoperative chemotherapy (100% vs. 63%). This is likely a surrogate for a perceived more aggressive initial clinical presentation. Similarly, Wicherts et al. [30] found that multiple preoperative lines of chemotherapy predicted failure to complete both stages.

While the data are still limited, morbidity and mortality rates of two-stage hepatectomy are comparable to population-based estimates reported after one-stage hepatectomy and, not surprisingly, are associated with the extent of resection. In fact, the incidence and severity of postoperative complications are generally lower after the first operation than following the second stage of hepatic resection. In particular, in the largest published series, investigators noted that none of the first-stage complications was major, in contrast to 33% of the postoperative complicating events considered major after the second hepatectomy [30]. Similarly, postoperative deaths have, in most cases, followed the second, major hepatectomy. Yet, more recently, the systematic use of PVE or PVL resulted in a reduced incidence of postoperative hepatic insufficiency and fatalities.

Table 8.1 Technical aspects, short- and long-term outcomes following two-stage hepatectomy

Author	Year	Patients (n)	Completion rate	PVE/PVL	Interval 1st-2nd stage (months)	Morbidity 1st stage (%)	Morbidity 2nd stage (%)	Mortality 1st stage (%)	Mortality 2nd stage (%)	OS 3-years (%)	OS 5-years (%)	Recurrence rate (%)
Adam [24]	2000	16	81%	6/0	4 (2–14)	43	54	0	15.4	35	–	69
Jaeck [25]	2004	33	76%	33/0	–	15	56	0	0	54.4	–	64
Chun [31]	2007	30	70%	12/0	2 (1.2–16)	24	43	0	0	86	–	54
Pachema [34]	2008	14	78%	5/0	7 (3–14)	0	27	0	0	–	50	72
Wicherts [30]	2008	59	69%	32/0	3.3 (1–15.7)	7	29	0	7	60	42	49
Mentha [35]	2009	23	95.6%	8/5	1–2	18	23	0	0	63	24	82
Tsai [32]	2010	45	78%	3/32	4.5 (2–22)	26	26	4	5	58	–	62
Karoui [28]	2010	33[a]	76%	5/17	3.7 (1.3–12)	21	32	0	4	80	48	62

PVE, Portal Vein Embolization; *PVL*, Portal Vein Ligature

[a]Included only patients with concomitant colorectal resection

Although early reports of survival after two-stage hepatectomy were initially modest, more recent series have reported 3-year overall survival estimates ranging from 54% to 60 % (Table 8.1). The most mature experiences reported cumulative 5-year survivals of 42% [30] and 48% [28], with a median follow-up of 24.4 and 28.7 months, respectively. Importantly, despite an initial presentation with bilateral, multifocal liver metastases, patients who successfully completed the two-stage approach had an overall survival comparable to that of patients who underwent a planned single-stage hepatectomy [31, 32]. Moreover, the recurrence rate, which was approximately 62% (Table 8.1), was not dissimilar to the 56% reported after single-stage hepatectomies [33]. Interestingly, Jaeck et al. [25] observed that the combination of resection and radiofrequency ablation increased the feasibility of two-stage hepatectomy by 20% (5 of 25 patients), with similar overall and disease-free survival as in patients undergoing liver resection alone. However, local ablation should be used only when resection alone does not allow for complete tumor clearance without jeopardizing the integrity of the FLR.

This surgical approach to multinodular and bilobar metastatic disease, almost always preceded by induction chemotherapy, has rapidly obtained widespread diffusion. It permits expansion of the pool of surgical candidates and optimizes patient selection for aggressive treatment, while morbidity is minimized.

8.4
Interstitial Treatments

Many patients with colorectal liver metastases are not candidates for resection of all the hepatic disease because of the presence of liver malignancy in unresectable locations, the number and anatomic distribution of tumor lesions, the presence of extrahepatic disease that is unresectable, and/or poor liver function. To compliment resectional strategies when complete resection of all metastases is not possible, a number of tumor ablative techniques have been explored, including radiofrequency ablation (RFA), microwave ablation (MWA), and cryosurgical ablation (CSA).

8.4.1
Interstitial Treatments Associated with Liver Resection

Ablative therapy in unresectable colorectal liver metastases has been used in combination with hepatic resections, in which hepatectomy addresses the main tumor mass and the residual tumor that cannot be resected is treated with local tumor-ablative therapy (Fig. 8.3). These strategies increase the number of patients who are eligible for aggressive surgical removal or destruction of their tumors. An international multi-institutional series [36] of patients treated with colorectal liver metastases reported that RFA was used in conjunction with resection in 8.0% of the 1669 patients in the study.

8 Therapeutic Strategies in Unresectable Colorectal Liver Metastases

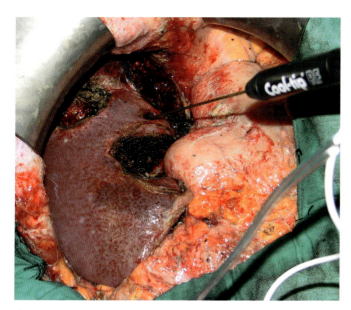

Fig. 8.3 Wedge resection associated with radiofrequency ablation of unresectable, centrally located, recurrent liver metastases 2 years after a left hepatectomy

In 2003, Pawlik et al. [37] reported on the largest series of patients (172) to have been treated simultaneously with hepatic resection and RFA. In this study, the rates of morbidity (19.8%) and mortality (2.3%) were comparable to those for hepatic resection alone. RFA of a tumor > 3 cm in diameter was a significant factor on multivariate analysis, with these patients having a higher likelihood of death from cancer recurrence than those who underwent ablation of a lesion < 3 cm. Patients who had RFA of a lesion > 3 cm showed a trend toward worse survival. In 2007, Abdalla et al. [38] published the results obtained in patients with non-resectable disease who were treated with RFA (alone or plus resection) vs. those who underwent the gold standard of resection. The only detectable difference between the groups was in the anatomic distribution of the tumors, which made complete resection impossible in the RFA groups. Despite comparable characteristics of traditional predictors, resection resulted in significantly better overall survival. The 4-year survival after resection ($n = 190$), RFA plus resection ($n = 101$), and RFA only ($n = 57$) was 65%, 36%, and 22%, respectively. Sub-analysis of patients with solitary lesions showed similar results. Survival differences appeared to be associated with a significantly higher intrahepatic failure rate and a higher true local recurrence rate after RFA.

Tanaka et al. [39] analyzed retrospectively 53 patients with five or more bilobar liver metastases from colorectal cancer who underwent hepatectomy with (16 patients) or without (37 patients) microwave ablation. A planned two-stage hepatectomy was carried out in 38% of the patients in both groups. Although the disease stage was advanced and the extent of hepatectomy tended to be smaller in patients with resection/ablation, no significant differences were found for overall, disease-free, or hepatic recurrence-free survival between the two groups. The authors suggested that microwave ablation plus hepatic resection allows the indications for hepatic resection to be extended to five or more bilobar liver metastases.

8.4.2
Interstitial Treatments Alone

8.4.2.1
Radiofrequency Ablation

At present, thermal ablation alone is used to treat metastatic liver disease in patients who are not candidates for surgical resection because of a medical inability to undergo resection or because they have tumors that are unresectable by virtue of their number, location, or size relative to liver volume.

RFA can be performed at open laparotomy, by laparoscopic surgery, or percutaneously. Radiofrequency electrodes are guided into position by ultrasound, CT, or MRI guidance and ablation is monitored by similar imaging modalities. During open and laparoscopic RFA, adjacent organs can easily be protected from burn injuries. The advantages of percutaneous techniques are: less surgical trauma, shorter hospital stay, and lower costs. It is also easier to repeat percutaneous treatment in case of residual tumor or recurrence. Its main disadvantage is that it is less reliable, especially for larger lesions and superficial lesions. For all approaches, correct positioning of the RFA probe is crucial, which requires experience and skill. For example, Poon et al. described a clear learning curve for RFA, percutaneously as well as surgically [40]. In their first 50 patients, complete tumor ablation was achieved in 85%, with most of the incomplete ablations in percutaneously treated patients, whereas in the next 50 patients 100% tumor ablation was accomplished.

Efficacy

The main factor influencing the efficacy of RFA is tumor size. For tumors < 2.5 cm, a technically successful ablation is possible in more than 90% of cases; in tumors between 2.5 and 3.5 cm the rate is 70–90%, and in tumors between 3.5 cm and 5 cm, 50–70%; however, for metastases > 5 cm the rate of successful ablation is less than 50% [41]. In the literature, local recurrence rates range from 1.8% to 39% [42, 43]. A meta-analysis of the local recurrence rate after hepatic RFA was recently published by Mulier et al. [44]. Their series comprised hepatocellular carcinoma (2369 lesions), unspecified lesions (1046), and colon cancer metastases (763 lesions). In multivariate analysis, significantly less local recurrences were observed for small size lesions ($p < 0.001$) and for lesions treated by a surgical (vs. percutaneous) approach ($p < 0.001$).

Complications

RFA is a relatively safe procedure with a low mortality rate (0–2%) and a low major complication rate [45]. Complication rates (major and minor) vary widely in the published literature (based primarily on the RFA approach). The range of reported complications rates is between 0 and 30.7%, with rates of 6–9% most commonly reported [45].

Long-term Results

Oshowo et al. [46] reported on a comparative series of patients with solitary colorectal metastases treated by RFA or hepatectomy. Although their study found similar 3-year survival rates in the two groups (53% for RFA and 55% for liver resection), it is striking that there were no long-term survivors following hepatectomy. These results conflict with well-established data showing 10- and 20-year survivors after hepatectomy of solitary and multiple metastases, even without adjuvant chemotherapy [47]. They also strongly contradict the results published by Aloi et al. [48]. In their series of patients with solitary liver metastasis as the first metastatic site treated for cure by hepatic resection or RFA, the survival rate following hepatic resection exceeded 70% at 5 years. Besides, RFA for solitary metastasis is associated with a markedly higher liver recurrence rate and shorter recurrence-free and overall survival, even when small lesions (< 3 cm) are considered. Similar results were reported by Reuter et al. [49] in a retrospective review of 66 patients who underwent RFA and 126 who underwent hepatectomy. Nevertheless, the two groups were similar based on Fong score and mean number of hepatic lesions; median time to recurrence was shorter with ablation than with resection. Recurrence at the ablation/resection site and distant recurrence were more common after ablation than after resection. In a recent study, Otto et al. [50] compared 28 patients with colorectal liver metastases detected within the first year after colorectal surgery treated by RFA with 82 patients who underwent liver resection for metastases not amenable to RFA due to number, size, or location. The median tumor size in patients treated by RFA was significantly lower. Nevertheless, local recurrence at the site of ablation or resection occurred in 32% and 4% ($p < 0.001$) respectively, while time to progression was significantly shorter in patients primarily treated with RFA (203 vs. 416 days; $p = 0.017$).

8.4.2.2
Microwave Ablation

Microwave technology achieves higher intra-tumoral temperatures, larger ablative volumes, faster ablation times, improved convection profile, and less procedural pain than RFA [51]. The possible complications and limitations of MWA are similar to those of RFA, including biliary stenosis, formation of postoperative hepatic abscesses, and potential for damage to adjacent structures. Martin et al. [52] reported overall 90-day mortality and morbidity rates of 0% and 29%, respectively, from a cohort of 100 patients treated with a total of 270 MWAs. Only one patient developed a hepatic abscess, and there were no bleeding complications. In this phase II study, recurrence at the ablation site occurred in 6% of patients with a median size of liver metastases ablated of 3 cm. Median disease-free survival for patients with liver colorectal metastases was 12 months, with an overall survival of 36 months.

8.4.2.3
Cryoablation

Newer thermal ablation modalities, including RFA and MWA, have more or less replaced CSA in the management of colorectal liver metastases. Local recurrence, which should be interpreted as a direct failure of cryotherapy, is observed in 0–22% of the cases [53, 54], although a local recurrence rate as high as 44% has been reported [55]. Local recurrence is mostly due to large tumor size, inadequate ultrasound monitoring, use of an inadequate probe diameter, or cryotherapy of lesions situated close to large vessels. Most series on cryosurgery report a mortality rate below 5% [56]. Acute post-operative myocardial infarction is the most common cause of death, followed by cryoshock and pulmonary complications. The latter include chest infection and atelectasis, occur in up to 25% of the patients, and are generally related to upper abdominal surgery. Pleural effusion is often encountered, but is generally transient and does not require drainage. Hemorrhage during or after the freezing process is seen in up to 9% of the patients and is mostly caused by cracking of the ice ball [56].

Weaver et al. [57] reported on 136 patients with unresectable colorectal liver metastases, which varied in number from 1 to 10. The 2- and 5-year survival rates in the study were 62% and 20%, respectively, and the median survival was 30 months. In a recent study of Xu et al. [58], 326 patients with non-resectable hepatic colorectal metastases underwent percutaneous CSA under the guidance of ultrasound or CT. During a median follow-up of 36 months (7–62 months), the median survival of all patients was 29 months (range 3–62 months). The recurrence rate was 47.2% during a median follow-up of 32 months (range 7–61). Among the recurrences, 61% were seen in the liver only and 13.9% in the liver and in extrahepatic areas. The recurrence rate at the cryotreated site was 6.4% for all cases.

At present, there is no evidence that interstitial treatments are equal to resection, mainly for local recurrences, and a randomized study of interstitial treatments vs. liver resection cannot ethically be supported at this time. Until such proof, resection of liver metastases remains the gold standard.

References

1. Abdalla EK, Hicks ME, Vauthey JN (2001) Portal vein embolization: rationale, technique, future prospects. Br J Surg 88:165–175
2. Imamura H, Shimada R, Kubota M et al (1999) Preoperativeportal vein embolization: an audit of 84 patients. Hepatology 29:1099–1105
3. Azoulay D, Castaing D, Smail A et al (2000) Resection of nonresectable liver metastases from colorectal cancer after percutaneousportal vein embolization. Ann Surg 231:480–486
4. Ferrero A, Viganò L, Polastri R et al (2007) Postoperative Liver Dysfunction and Future Remnant Liver: Where Is the Limit? Results of a Prospective Study. World J Surg 31:1643–1651
5. Di Stefano DR, de Baere T, Denys A et al (2005) Preoperative Percutaneous Portal Vein Embolization: Evaluation of Adverse Events in 188 Patients. Radiology 234:625–630
6. Broering DC, Hillert C, Krupski G et al (2002) Portal Vein Embolization vs. Portal Vein Ligation for Induction of Hypertrophy of the Future Liver Remnant. J Gastrointest Surg 6:905–913
7. Capussotti L, Muratore A, Baracchi F et al (2008) Portal Vein Ligation as an Efficient Method of Increasing the Future Liver Remnant Volume in the Surgical Treatment of Colorectal Metastases. Arch Surg 143:978-982
8. Abulkhir A, Limongelli P, Healey AJ et al (2008) Preoperative Portal Vein Embolization for Major Liver Resection. A Meta-Analysis. Ann Surg 247:49–57
9. Capussotti L, Muratore A, Ferrero A et al (2005) Extension of Right Portal Vein Embolization to Segment IV Portal Branches. Arch Surg 140:1100-1103
10. Ribero D, Abdalla EK, Madoff DC et al (2007) Portal vein embolization before major hepatectomy and its effects on regeneration, resectability and outcome. Br J Surg 94:1386-94
11. de Graaf W, van den Esschert JW, van Lienden KP et al (2009) Induction of tumor growth after preoperative portal vein embolization: is it a real problem? Ann Surg Oncol 16:423-30
12. Elias D, De Baere T, Roche A et al (1999) During liver regeneration following right portal embolization the growth rate of liver metastases is more rapid than that of the liver parenchyma. Br J Surg 86:784-8
13. Kokudo N, Tada K, Seki M, Ohta H et al (2001) Proliferative activity of intrahepatic colorectal metastases after preoperative hemihepatic portal vein embolization. Hepatology 34:267-72
14. Di Stefano G, Derenzini M, Kratz F et al (2004) Liver-targeted doxorubicin: effects on rat regenerating hepatocytes. Liver Int 24:246–252
15. Goere D, Farges O, Leporrier J et al (2006) Chemotherapy Does Not Impair Hypertrophy of the Left Liver After Right Portal Vein Obstruction. J Gastrointest Surg 10:365–370
16. Zorzi D, Chun YS, Madoff DC et al (2008) Chemotherapy with bevacizumab does not affect liver regeneration after portal vein embolization in the treatment of colorectal liver metastases. Ann Surg Oncol 15:2765-72
17. Aussilhou B, Dokmak S, Faivre S et al (2009) Preoperative liver hypertrophy induced by portal flow occlusion before major hepatic resection for colorectal metastases can be impaired by bevacizumab.Ann Surg Oncol 16:1553-9
18. Hemming AW, Reed AI, Howard RJ et al (2003) Preoperative portal vein embolization for extended hepatectomy. Ann Surg 237:686-91
19. Wicherts DA, de Haas RJ, Andreani P et al (2010) Impact of portal vein embolization on long-term survival of patients with primarily unresectable colorectal liver metastases. Br J Surg 97:240-50
20. Pamecha V, Glantzounis G, Davies N et al (2009) Long-term survival and disease recurrence following portal vein embolisation prior to major hepatectomy for colorectal metastases. Ann Surg Oncol 16:1202-7

21. Oussoultzoglou E, Bachellier P, Rosso E et al (2006) Right portal vein embolization before right hepatectomy for unilobar colorectal liver metastases reduces the intrahepatic recurrence rate. Ann Surg 244:71-79

22. Abdalla EK, Adam R, Bilchik AJ et al (2006) Improving resectability of hepatic colorectal metastases: expert consensus statement. Ann Surg Oncol 13:1271-1280

23. Scheele J, Stangl R, Altendorf-Hofmann A (1990) Hepatic metastases from colorectal carcinoma: impact of surgical resection on the natural history. Br J Surg 77:1241–1246

24. Adam R, Laurent A, Azoulay D, et al (2000) Two-stage hepatectomy: a planed strategy to treat irresectable liver tumors. Ann Surg 232:777–785

25. Jaeck D, Oussoultzoglou E, Rosso E et al (2004) A two-stage hepatectomy with portal vein embolization to achieve curative resection for initially unresectable and bilobar colorectal liver metastases. Ann Surg 240:1037–1051

26. Thelen A, Jonas S, Benckert C et al (2007) Simultaneous versus staged liver resection of synchronous liver metastases from colorectal cancer. Int J Colorectal Dis 22:1269-1276

27. Reddy SK, Pawlik TM, Zorzi D et al (2007) Simultaneous resections of colorectal cancer and synchronous liver metastases: a multi-institutional analysis. Ann Surg Oncol 14:3481-3491

28. Karoui M, Viganò L, Tayar C et al (2010) Combined first stage hepatectomy at the time of colorectal resection in two-stage hepatectomy procedures for patients with bilobar synchronous liver metastases. Br J Surg, in press

29. Tanaka K, Shimada H, Matsuo K et al (2007) Regeneration after two-stage hepatectomy vs repeat resection for colorectal metastasis recurrence. J Gastrointest Surg 11:1154-1161

30. Wicherts DA, Miller R, de Haas RJ et al (2008) Long-term results of two-stage hepatecytomy for irresectable colorectal cancer liver metastases. Ann Surg 248:994-1005

31. Chun YS, Vauthey JN, Ribero D et al (2007) Systemic chemotherapy and two-stage hepatectomy for extensive bilateral colorectal liver metastases: perioperative safety and survival. J Gastrointest Surg 11:1498-1505

32. Tsai S, Marques HP, de Jong MC et al (2010) Two-stage strategy for patients with extensive bilateral colorectal liver metastases. HBP 12:262-269

33. de Jong MC, Pulitano C, Ribero D et al (2009) Rates and patterns of recurrence following curative intent surgery for colorectal liver metastasis. An international multi-institutional analysis of 1669 patients. Ann Surg 250:440–448

34. Pachema V, Nedjat-Shokouhi B, Gerusamy K et al (2008) Prospective evaluation of two-stage hepatectomy combined with selective portal vein embolisation and systemic chemotherapy for patients with unresectable colorectal liver metastases. Dig Surg 25:387-393

35. Mentha G, Terraz S, Morel P et al (2009) Dangerous halo after neoadjuvant chemotherapy and two-step hepatectomy for colorectal liver metastasis. Br J Surg 96:95-103

36. de Jong MC, Pulitano C, Ribero D et al (2009) Rates and patterns of recurrence following curative intent surgery for colorectal liver metastasis: an international multi-institutional analysis of 1669 patients. Ann Surg 250:440– 448

37. Pawlik TM, Izzo F, Cohen DS et al (2003) Combined Resection and Radiofrequency Ablation for Advanced Hepatic Malignancies: Results in 172 Patients. Ann Surg Oncol 10:1059-1069

38. Abdalla EK, Vauthey JN, Ellis Lm et al (2004) Recurrence and outcomes following hepatic resection, radiofrequency ablation, and combined resection/ablation for colorectal liver metastases. Ann Surg 239:818-825

39. Tanaka K, Shimada H, Nagano Y (2006) Outcome after hepatic resection versus combined resection and microwave ablation for multiple bilobar colorectal metastases to the liver. Surgery 139:263-273

40. Poon RT, Ng KK, Lam CM et al (2004) Learning curve for radiofrequency ablation of liver tumors: prospective analysis of initial 100 patients in a tertiary institution. Ann Surg 239: 441-449

8 Therapeutic Strategies in Unresectable Colorectal Liver Metastases

41. Solbiati L, Livraghi T, Goldberg SN et al (2001) Percutaneous radiofrequency ablation of hepatic metastases from colorectal cancer: Long-term results in 117 patients. Radiology 221:159–166
42. Bowles BJ, Machi J, Limm WL et al (2001) Safety and efficacy of radiofrequency thermal ablation in advanced liver tumors. Arch Surg 136:864–869
43. Siperstein A, Garland A, Engle K et al (2000) Local recurrence after laparoscopic radiofrequency thermal ablation of hepatic tumors. Ann Surg Oncol 7:106–113
44. Lewin JS, Connell CF, Duerk JL et al (1998) Interactive MRI-guided radiofrequency interstitial thermal ablation of abdominal tumors: Clinical trial for evaluation of safety and feasibility. J Magn Reson Imaging 8:40–47
45. Wong SL, Mangu PB, Choti MA et al (2010) American Society of Clinical Oncology 2009 Clinical Evidence Review on Radiofrequency Ablation of Hepatic Metastases From Colorectal Cancer. J Clinic Oncol 28:493-508
46. Oshowo A, Gillams A, Harrison E et al (2003) Comparison of resection and radiofrequency ablation for treatment of solitary colorectal liver metastases. Br J Surg 90:1240-1243
47. Scheele J, Stang R, Altendorf-Hofmann A et al (1995) Resection of colorectal liver metastases. World J Surg 19:59-71
48. Aloia TA, Vauthey JN, Loyer EM et al (2006) Solitary Colorectal Liver Metastasis Resection Determines Outcome. Arch Surg 141:460-466
49. Reuter NP, Woodall CE, Scoggins CR et al (2009) Radiofrequency Ablation vs. Resection for Hepatic Colorectal Metastasis: Therapeutically Equivalent? J Gastrointest Surg 13:486-491
50. Otto G, Düber C, Hoppe-Lotichius M et al (2010) Radiofrequency ablation as first-line treatment in patients with early colorectal liver metastases amenable to surgery. Ann Surg 251:796-803
51. Wright AS, Lee FT, Mahvi DM et al (2003) Hepatic microwave ablation with multiple antennae results in synergistically larger zones of coagulation necrosis. Ann Surg Oncol 10:275–283
52. Martin RC, Scoggins CR, McMasters KM et al (2007) Microwave hepatic ablation: initial experience of safety and efficacy. J Surg Oncol 96:481–486
53. Ravikumar TS, Kane R, Cady B et al (1991) A 5-year study of cryosurgery in the treatment of liver tumors. Arch Surg 126:1520-1524
54. Crews KA, Kuhn JA, McCarty TM et al (1997) Cryosurgical ablation of hepatic tumors. Am J Surg 174: 614-618
55. Adam R, Akpinar E, Johann M et al (1997) Place of cryosurgery in the treatment of malignant liver tumors. Ann Surg 225:39-50
56. Seifert JK, Junginger T, Morris DL (1998) A collective review of the world literature on hepatic cryotherapy. J R Coll Surg Edinb 43:141-143
57. Weaver ML, Ashton JG, Zemel R (1998) Treatment of colorectal liver metastases by cryotherapy. Sem Surg Oncol 14:163-170
58. Xu KC, Niu LZ, He WB, et al (2008) Percutaneous cryosurgery for the treatment of hepatic colorectal metastases. World J Gastroenterol 7:1430-1436

Extrahepatic Disease

9

Abstract The presence of extrahepatic disease synchronous to colorectal liver metastases was long considered a contraindication to resection. However, in recent series good survival rates after radical hepatic and extrahepatic resection have been reported and were higher than expected after chemotherapy alone. Portal lymph nodes involvement occurs in about 15% of patients and is a negative prognostic factor. Lymph node metastases confined to the hepatic pedicle are no longer a contraindication to resection, although preoperative chemotherapy is recommended. In patients with celiac or retroperitoneal positive lymph nodes, the indications for resection are controversial. Resection in the presence of peritoneal carcinomatosis should be considered only in well selected patients with limited resectable peritoneal deposits. Pulmonary metastases should be aggressively resected whenever possible, even if synchronous to liver metastases, as good long-term results are possible.

9.1
Introduction

Approximately 35% of patients affected by colorectal cancer have stage IV disease at diagnosis, i.e., metastatic disease, while 20–50% will develop metastases during follow-up. The most common sites of metastases are the liver, lung, and peritoneum. Liver and lung metastases are due to hematogenous tumor spread and occur in about 50% of patients with stage IV disease. Peritoneal carcinomatosis is caused by transmural spread of primary malignancy or by tumor perforation and occurs in about 10–25% of patients with recurrent disease. Other sites of metastases, including adrenal gland, bone, and brain, are uncommon and generally are seen at an advanced disease stage.

Early surgical experience regarding resection for colorectal liver metastases associated with extrahepatic disease (EHD) reported extremely poor outcomes for these patients [1-3]. Based on these data, the presence of associated EHD was long

---

R. Lo Tesoriere (✉)
Division of Hepato-Bilio-Pancreatic and Digestive Surgery, Mauriziano "Umberto I" Hospital, Turin, Italy

Surgical Treatment of Colorectal Liver Metastases. Lorenzo Capussotti (Ed.)
© Springer-Verlag Italia 2011

considered a contraindication to liver resection. However, recent improvements in surgical technique, preoperative staging accuracy, and chemotherapy effectiveness have led many authors to reconsider resection in this group of patients. Elias et al., in a study of 111 patients with EHD treated with resection, were one of the first to challenge EHD as a formal contraindication to surgery [4]. The most common sites of EHD in their series were peritoneum, lung, and local colorectal recurrence. After a median follow-up of 4.9 years, the 5-year overall survival rate was 20% vs. 34% in 265 patients with disease confined to the liver. Despite the negative prognostic value of EHD, patients who underwent resection had better survival results than those treated with chemotherapy alone. The same authors published a subsequent analysis in which only R0 resections were included [5]: 3- and 5-year overall survival rates in the presence of EHD were 45% and 28%, respectively, similar to those of patients undergoing R0 resection for liver-only metastases (56% and 33%, respectively). The authors concluded that EHD should no longer be considered an absolute contraindication to surgery, provided that radical resection is feasible. The largest clinical series of resections for colorectal liver metastases and simultaneous EHD was recently reported by Carpizo et al. [6]. In the 127 patients included in their study, the most common EHD sites were lung (26.8%) and hepatic pedicle lymph nodes (21.3%). The study patients were strictly selected: the majority of them had limited hepatic involvement (median number of metastases of 2) and EHD (1 site in 80.3% of patients). After a median follow-up of 24 months, the 5-year survival rate was 26% vs. 49% for patients without EHD ($p = 0.001$). Among patients with EHD, multivariate analysis identified the following prognostic factors: high clinical risk score [7], incomplete resection of EHD, intraoperatively detected EHD, and neoadjuvant chemotherapy. The authors concluded that the patients most likely to benefit from the resection of liver metastases and EHD are those with low clinical risk score and a single EHD deposit, in which complete resection can be achieved.

Thus, in summary, EHD simultaneous to liver metastases is no longer an absolute contraindication to resection. However, the EHD site has a significant impact on prognosis and surgical indications. The most common sites of EHD are considered separately in the following pages.

9.2
Lymph-node Metastases

Perihepatic lymph-node (LN) involvement in patients with colorectal liver metastases represents the locoregional spread of metastatic tumors through the lymphatics (Fig. 9.1). Even if supradiaphragmatic lymphatic drainage has been reported in anatomic studies, the most common sites of LN metastases are along the hepatic pedicle, the common hepatic artery, the celiac trunk, and the retropancreatic area.

Recent studies, in which systematic LN dissection of the hepatic pedicle was performed, have assessed the real incidence of LN involvement. In 1997, Beckurts et al. reported on a series of 126 patients undergoing liver resection for colorectal metas-

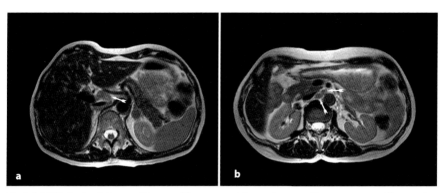

Fig. 9.1 MRI obtained from a 52-year-old woman with synchronous liver metastases from a sigmoid adenocarcinoma and intra-abdominal lymph node metastases confirmed by PET/CT. **a** A 2.3-cm hepatic pedicle lymph node (*arrow*). **b** Metastatic para-aortic lymph nodes (*arrows*), which contraindicated liver resection

tases and systematic hepatic pedicle LN dissection [8]. The incidence of LN metastases was 28%. In a similar study by Elias et al. [9], microscopic LN metastases were demonstrated in 14% of 114 consecutive patients. The occurrence of LN metastases was significantly associated with the number of liver metastases (≥ 3), the CEA value (> 118 ng/ml), and the extent of liver involvement by the tumor (> 15%). Similar data were reported by Laurent et al. (15%) [10] and Ercolani et al. (14%) [11]. All of the authors concluded that, due to the frequency of LN metastases, LN dissection should be regularly performed as a staging procedure during any liver resection for metastases. However, the indications for LN dissection are still debated. Recently, Grobmyer et al. [12] analyzed the contribution of preoperative imaging and intraoperative assessment to the detection of portal LN metastases in 100 patients undergoing resection for primary and secondary hepatic malignancies. Among patients with no suspicion of LN involvement, neither at CT nor at PET-CT, nor at intraoperative palpation, none (0 out of 39) had LN metastases. This study confirms that imaging and intraoperative palpation can detect almost all LN metastases and that routine LN dissection is not justified. Thus, further studies are needed to clarify the indications for LN dissection.

The presence of LN metastases is an established negative prognostic factor. The outcomes of patients undergoing resection for colorectal liver metastases and concurrent portal LN metastases are summarized in Table 9.1. In early studies, the presence of positive LN was associated with extremely poor outcomes and was considered a contraindication to surgery. In the above-mentioned series by Beckurts et al. [8], the 5-year survival rate in LN-positive patients was 0% compared to 22% in LN-negative ones. These data were confirmed by Laurent et al. (5-year survival rates 5% vs. 43%) [10]. However, many biases affected these studies: they were retrospective analyses, included few patients, usually considered palpable macroscopic LN metastases, and were carried out in an era predating modern chemotherapy regimens and imaging. In 2002, Jaeck et al. [13] strongly contributed to the debate concerning surgical indica-

Table 9.1 Outcomes of patients undergoing resection for colorectal liver metastases and concurrent portal lymph-node metastases (*LN*)

	LN + patients	Overall survival LN+		Overall survival LN-			Prognostic factor
		3 years (%)	5 years (%)	3 years (%)	5 years (%)	p	
Ekberg (1986) [16]	6/68 (9%)	10	0	36	20	0.01	Y
Rosen (1992) [17]	9/271 (3%)	11	0	48	25	0.002	Y
Beckurts (1997) [8]	35/126 (28%)	3	0	48	22	0.0001	Y
Minagawa (2000) [18]	6/235 (3%)	0	0	52	39	0.0001	Y
Jaeck (2002) [13]	17/160 (11%)	19	0	62	47	0.001	Y
Laurent (2004) [10]	23/156 (15%)	27	5	56	43	0.0001	Y
Bennett (2008) [19]	8/59 (14%)	25	NR	75	NR	0.045	Y
Adam (2008) [14]	47/763 (6%)	15	11	34	23	0.004	Y
Oussoultzoglou (2009) [15]	45/NR	29.3	17.3	NR	NR	NR	NR

NR, Not reported; *Y*, yes

tions in LN-positive patients. The authors prospectively performed systematic LN dissection in 160 patients and assessed the prognostic impact of the presence and location of LN metastases. LN-positive patients (17 out of 160, 11%) had worse survival than LN-negative ones (3-year overall survival rates 19% vs. 62%, respectively). LN-positive patients were further stratified according to the sites of their LN metastases. Patients with celiac LN metastases had significantly worse survival than those with LN metastases in the hepatic pedicle (3-year overall survival rates 0% vs. 38%). According to these data, only LN metastases in the celiac area should be considered a contraindication to surgery, while LN involvement confined to the hepatic pedicle should not preclude resection. The impact of neoadjuvant chemotherapy on the prognostic role of LN metastases was recently considered. Adam et al. [14] reviewed the outcomes of 47 patients with LN metastases, either portal, celiac, or retroperitoneal, representing 6% of the series of 763 patients resected for liver metastases. All 47 patients received preoperative chemotherapy, which always led to LN disease response or stabilization. The 5-year overall survival rate was 18% in the LN-positive group vs. 53% in the LN-negative one (p = 0.001). According to the LN deposit site, the 5-year overall survival rate was 25% in the hepatic pedicle LN group, 0% in the celiac group, and 0% in the para-aortic group (p = 0.001). The authors concluded that chemotherapy response should not modify indications; that is, hepatectomy with LN dissection is justified in patients with regional LN involvement, while patients with either celiac or para-aortic LN metastases (Fig. 9.1b) should not be scheduled for resection, even if they respond to preoperative chemotherapy. Different results were recently reported by the Strasbourg group [15], who analyzed a series of 45 patients with LN metastases receiving extensive pre- and/or postoperative chemotherapy (53% and 80% of cases, respectively). The 5-year survival rate was 25.7% in patients with hepatic pedicle LN involvement and 16.7% in patients with common hepatic artery and celiac trunk LN involvement (p = n.s.). Similar disease-free survival rates were also observed. At multivariate analysis, CEA level before hepatectomy, R0 liver resection, involved/dissected LN ratio, and adjuvant chemotherapy administration were significant prognostic factors. In the chemotherapy era, the prognostic role of LN metastases site remains controversial. Further studies are needed to clarify whether chemotherapy could enlarge the surgical indications to include patients with LN metastases outside the hepatic pedicle.

9.3
Peritoneal Carcinomatosis

Peritoneal carcinomatosis (PC) from colorectal cancer occurs by tumor invading through the full-thickness bowel wall, by rupture of non-invasive tumor, or by intraperitoneal spread during surgical procedures. Between 13% and 25% of patients with recurrent colorectal cancer develop synchronous or metachronous peritoneal metastases (Fig. 9.2). Traditionally, PC was considered a contraindication to surgery but localized PC is no longer viewed as systemic dissemination of disease, but rather

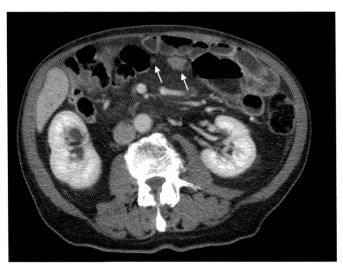

Fig. 9.2 CT scan obtained from a 67-year-old man with metachronous liver metastases and peritoneal carcinomatosis. *Arrows* indicate two peritoneal implants

as regional spread. Jayne et al. [20] reported that PC is localized in 64% of patients. This finding has provided the rationale for treating localized PC by resection and intraperitoneal chemotherapy. There are many retrospective studies [21] and one randomized clinical trial [22] reporting improved survival rates after combined cytoreductive surgery (CRS) and perioperative intraperitoneal chemotherapy (PIC) vs. palliative chemotherapy. Nonetheless, published results should be interpreted in the context of extreme selection bias and cannot be generalized to all patients with colorectal PC.

In most series, extraperitoneal disease has been considered a contraindication to surgical treatment in patients with PC [23, 24], and PC a contraindication in those with potentially resectable liver metastases. Recently, some cases of simultaneous treatment of liver metastases and PC have been published. Elias et al. [25] evaluated 24 patients with moderate PC and liver metastases undergoing CRS, PIC, and liver resection (including six major hepatectomies). There was one postoperative death and the morbidity rate was 58%. The 3-year survival rate was 41.5%. Kianmanesh et al. [26] analyzed 43 patients treated for colorectal cancer PC, including 16 with liver metastases. Median survival was similar in patients with or without associated liver metastases (36.0 vs. 35.3 months). A multicenter French study [27] recently reported the largest series of CRS and PIC for PC: 523 patients from 23 centers, including 77 patients with liver metastases. Overall mortality and severe morbidity rates were 3% and 31%, respectively. After a median follow-up of 45 months, 5-year overall and disease-free survival rates were 27% and 10%, respectively. The extent of PC and the presence of LN metastases were significant negative prognostic factors, while the presence of liver metastases was not. In the analysis of 416 patients undergoing complete treatment (no macroscopic residual cancer), the presence of liver metastases

9 Extrahepatic Disease

achieved a negative impact on survival, together with PC extent and LN status. The authors concluded that the presence of liver metastases associated with extensive PC should be considered a contraindication to treatment.

9.4
Pulmonary Metastases

The liver and the lung are the two most common sites of distant metastases from colorectal cancer. The role of surgical treatment for colorectal pulmonary metastases has been established. There is a substantial body of evidence from retrospective series demonstrating that resection of colorectal pulmonary metastases can be safely performed, with low mortality (0–2.5%) and good survival results in selected patients. Reported 5-year overall survival rates range between 24% and 64% [28, 29].

Unfortunately, most studies considered isolated pulmonary resection and few data are available regarding combined liver and pulmonary resections. Miller et al. [30] reported on a series of 131 patients with colorectal cancer who underwent resection of hepatic and pulmonary metastases over a 20-year period. The site of first metastasis was the liver in 85 patients (65%), the lung in 14 (11%), and the liver and lung simultaneously in 32 (24%) patients. Thus, the liver was involved as a component of the first metastatic episode in 89% of patients. The authors reported 5-year survival rates of 49% after resection of the first metastasis, 48% after resection of liver metastases, and 31% after resection of both sites. These results must be interpreted in the context of a high selection bias, as confirmed by pathological data showing that the median number of liver and lung metastases was 2 and 1, respectively. No predefined algorithms were followed in patient selection and the resection decision relied only on the surgeon's case-by-case evaluation. Except for one French study (43 patients, 5-year survival rate of 11%) [31], all the other reports have confirmed the good long-term outcomes achieved after the resection of hepatic and pulmonary metastases (30%–74%) [32-34].

Many studies have tried to identify prognostic factors in order to select good candidates for surgery. Synchronous presentation of liver and lung metastases has been reported to negatively impact survival [35, 36], as well as a short disease-free interval between the first and second metastasectomy (liver or lung) [30] and the presence of multiple pulmonary nodules [33] (Fig. 9.3). At present, no clear guidelines are available for patient selection. Published studies concerning the resection of hepatic and lung metastases from colorectal cancer are summarized in Table 9.2.

The sequence of resection in patients who present with resectable simultaneous liver and lung metastases should be individualized. Although simultaneous resection is feasible in selected patients, in most cases it is preferable to have the patient recover from one operation before proceeding with the other, especially in technically challenging procedures. The choice of the initial procedure, laparotomy or thoracotomy, should depend on which one has the highest likelihood of revealing unresectable disease.

Table 9.2 Published retrospective studies of patients undergoing resection for colorectal cancer metastatic to the liver and lungs

	Patients (n)	Liver-lung synchronous metastases	Liver-lung metachronous metastases	5-year OS[a]	Prognostic factors of OS
Kobayashi (1999) [33]	47	21	26	31%	Solitary vs. multiple pulmonary metastases
Nagakura (2001) [35]	27	10	17	27%[b]	Metachronous vs. synchronous Age at first metastasectomy (> 60 years)
Mineo (2003) [36]	29	12	17	51%	Metachronous vs. synchronous Elevated CEA and CA19-9 level
Reddy (2004) [37]	26	5	21	50%[c]	NR
Shah (2006) [34]	39	11	28	74%[b]	None
Miller (2007) [30]	131	32	99	32%[d]	Age > 55 years Multiple metastases Disease-free interval between first and second metastasis < 1 year
Neef (2009) [38]	44	7	37	27%	First metastasis lung vs. liver

NR, Not Reported; *OS*, Overall Survival

[a]From last metastasectomy

[b]5-year overall survival reported from the first metastasectomy

[c]3-year survival

[d]Disease-specific survival

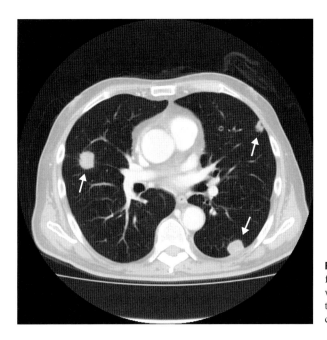

Fig. 9.3 CT scan obtained from a 46-year-old man with bilateral lung metastases (*arrows*) from a rectal cancer

9.5 Other Sites

9.5.1 Locoregional Recurrence

Primary rectal tumors are associated with a higher risk of locoregional recurrence as compared to colonic lesions. The local recurrence rate following rectal surgery ranges from 3% to 30%. No study has specifically addressed the treatment of local recurrences associated with liver metastases. A small number of cases (3–15%) [4, 6, 39] are included in most studies of EHD; thus, because of the sample size, specific analyses are not possible. However, primary tumor recurrence associated with liver metastases, when radically resectable, does not represent a contraindication to liver resection.

9.5.2 Adrenal Metastases

Adrenal metastases (AM) from colorectal cancer generally occur at an advanced disease stage. Solitary AM are rare, with a total of 14 papers reporting 36 patients undergoing adrenalectomy. AM synchronous to liver metastases have been rarely reported in the literature. A recent retrospective French study [40] analyzed this specific issue, comparing the outcomes of patients treated for both liver metastases and AM (diagnosed pre-, intra- and post-operatively) with those of patients treated for liver-only disease. Fourteen (1.8%) out of 796 patients had associated AM: ten underwent resection, while four were not operated on because of unresectable disease. Survival was significantly lower in the AM group (at 5 years from diagnosis 32% vs. 53%, $p = 0.02$). For the 14 patients with AM, median survival after diagnosis was 23 months and was similar whether they were treated by adrenalectomy plus chemotherapy or by chemotherapy alone. However, one patient who underwent resection survived more than 7 years. The prognostic significance of AM remains unclear.

9.5.3
Bone and Brain Metastases

Metastases of colorectal cancer to bones are very uncommon, involving less than 10% of patients. Their onset is usually late in the natural history of the cancer, is almost constantly preceded by liver and/or lung metastases, and often indicates the terminal phase of the disease. Brain metastases are even less common and equally indicative of terminal stage disease. For these reasons, bone and brain metastases are, at present, formal contraindication to surgical treatment.

9.6
Conclusions

The presence of EHD synchronous to colorectal liver metastases was long considered a contraindication to resection. However, recent series have reported good survival rates after radical hepatic and extrahepatic resection, higher than expected after chemotherapy alone. Portal lymph nodes involvement occurs in about 15% of patients and is a negative prognostic factor. Lymph node metastases confined to the hepatic pedicle are no longer a contraindication to resection, although preoperative chemotherapy is recommended. In patients with celiac or retroperitoneal positive lymph nodes, indications for resection are still controversial. Resection in the presence of peritoneal carcinomatosis should be considered only in well selected patients with limited resectable peritoneal deposits. Pulmonary metastases should be aggressively resected whenever possible, even if synchronous to liver metastases, because good long-term results are possible. The current indications for resection of extrahepatic disease are summarized in Table 9.3.

9 Extrahepatic Disease

Table 9.3 Summary of the current indications for resection of extrahepatic disease. In all cases, surgery is indicated only if complete resection can be achieved

Indications in the presence of extrahepatic disease	
Abdominal localization	
Lymph-node metastases	
Hepatic pedicle	Resection
Celiac	Contraindication
	Debated, if response to chemotherapy
Para-aortic	Contraindication
Peritoneal carcinomatosis	Resection if limited
Colorectal recurrence	Resection
Adrenal metastases	Debated
Extra-abdominal localization	
Lung	Resection
Bone	Contraindication
Brain	Contraindication

References

1. Cady B, McDermott WV (1985) Major hepatic resection for metachronous metastases from colon cancer. Ann Surg 210: 204-209
2. Foster JH (1978) Survival after liver resection for secondary tumors. Am J Surg 135:389-394
3. Adson MA (1989) The resection of hepatic metastases. Another view. Arch Surg 124:1023-1024
4. Elias D, Ouellet JF, Bellon N et al (2003) Extrahepatic disease does not contraindicate hepatectomy for colorectal liver metastases. Br J Surg 90:567-574
5. Elias D, Sideris L, Pocard M et al (2004) Results of R0 resection for colorectal liver metastases associated with extrahepatic disease. Ann Surg Oncol 11:274-280
6. Carpizo DR, Are C, Jarnagin W et al (2009) Liver resection for metastatic colorectal cancer in patients with concurrent extrahepatic disease: results in 127 patients treated at a single center. Ann Surg Oncol 16:2138-2146
7. Fong Y, Fortner J, Sun RL et al (1999) Clinical score for predicting recurrence after hepatic resection for metastatic colorectal cancer: analysis of 1001 consecutive cases. Ann Surg 230: 309-318
8. Beckurts KT, Holscher AH, Thorban S et al (1997) Significance of lymph node involvement at the hepatic hilum in the resection of colorectal liver metastases. Br J Surg 84:1081-1084
9. Elias D, Saric J, Jaeck D et al (1996) Prospective study of microscopic lymph node involvement of the hepatic pedicle during curative hepatectomy for colorectal metastases. Br J Surg 83:942-945
10. Laurent C, Sa Cunha A, Rullier E et al (2004) Impact of microscopic hepatic lymph node involvement on survival after resection of colorectal liver metastasis. J Am Coll Surg 198:884-891

11. Ercolani G, Grazi GL, Ravaioli M et al (2004) The role of lymphadenectomy for liver tumors: further considerations on the appropriateness of treatment strategy. Ann Surg 239:202-209

12. Grobmyer SR, Wang L, Gonen M et al (2006) Perihepatic lymph node assessment in patients undergoing partial hepatectomy for malignancy. Ann Surg 244: 260-264

13. Jaeck D, Nakano H, Bachellier P et al (2002) Significance of hepatic pedicle lymph node involvement in patients with colorectal liver metastases: a prospective study. Ann Surg Oncol 9:430-438

14. Adam R, de Haas RJ, Wicherts DA et al (2008) Is hepatic resection justified after chemotherapy in patients with colorectal liver metastases and lymph node involvement? J Clin Oncol 26:3672–3680

15. Oussoultzoglou E, Romain B, Panaro F et al (2009) Long-term survival after liver resection for colorectal liver metastases in patients with hepatic pedicle lymph nodes involvement in the era of new chemotherapy regimens. Ann Surg 249:879-886

16. Ekberg H, Tranberg KG, Andersson R et al (1986) Determinants of survival in liver resection for colorectal secondaries. Br J Surg 73:727-731

17. Rosen CB, Nagorney DM, Taswell HF et al (1992) Perioperative blood transfusion and determinants of survival after liver resection for metastatic colorectal carcinoma. Ann Surg 216:493-504

18. Minagawa M, Makuuchi M, Torzilli G et al (2000) Extension of the frontiers of surgical indications in the treatment of liver metastases from colorectal cancer: Long-term results. Ann Surg 231:487-499

19. Bennett JJ, Schmidt CR, Klimstra DS et al (2008) Perihepatic lymph node micrometastases impact outcome after partial hepatectomy for colorectal metastases. Ann Surg Oncol 15:1130-3116

20. Jayne DG, Fook S, Loi C et al (2002) Peritoneal carcinomatosis from colorectal cancer. Br J Surg 89:1545-1550

21. Yan TD, Black D, Savady R et al (2006) Systematic review on the efficacy of cytoreductive surgery combined with perioperative intraperitoneal chemotherapy for peritoneal carcinomatosis from colorectal carcinoma. J Clin Oncol 24:4011–4019

22. Verwaal VJ, van Ruth S, de Bree E et al (2003) Randomized trial of cytoreduction and hyperthermic intraperitoneal chemotherapy versus systemic chemotherapy and palliative surgery in patients with peritoneal carcinomatosis of colorectal cancer. J Clin Oncol 21:3737-3743

23. Sugarbaker PH (1998) Intraperitoneal chemotherapy and cytoreductive surgery for prevention and treatment of peritoneal carcinomatosis and sarcomatosis. Semin Surg Oncol 14:254-261

24. Glehen O, Kwiatkowski F, Sugarbaker PH et al (2004) Cytoreductive surgery combined with intraperitoneal chemotherapy for management of peritoneal carcinomatosis from colorectal cancer: a multi-institutional study J Clin Oncol 22:3284-3292

25. Elias D, Benizri E, Pocard M et al (2006) Treatment of synchronous peritoneal carcinomatosis and liver metastases from colorectal cancer. Eur J Surg Oncol 32:632-636

26. Kianmanesh R, Scaringi S, Sabate JM et al (2007) Iterative cytoreductive surgery associated with hyperthermic intraperitoneal chemotherapy for treatment of peritoneal carcinomatosis of colorectal origin with or without liver metastases. Ann Surg 245:597-603

27. Elias D, Gilly F, Boutitie F et al (2010) Peritoneal colorectal carcinomatosis treated with surgery and perioperative intraperitoneal chemotherapy: retrospective analysis of 523 patients from a multicentric french study. J Clin Oncol 28:63-68

28. Pfannschmidt J, Dienemann H, Hoffmann H (2007) Surgical resection of pulmonary metastases from colorectal cancer: a systematic review of published series. Ann Thorac Surg 84:324-338

29. Ashley AC, Deschamps C, Alberts SR (2006) Impact of prognostic factors on clinical outcome after resection of colorectal pulmonary metastases. Clin Colorectal Cancer 6:32–37

30. Miller G, Biernacki P, Kemeny NE et al (2007) Outcomes after resection of synchronous or metachronous hepatic and pulmonary colorectal metastases. J Am Coll Surg 205:231-238
31. Regnard JF, Grunenwald D, Spaggiari L et al (1998) Surgical treatment of hepatic and pulmonary metastases from colorectal cancers. Ann Thorac Surg 66:214-218
32. Headrick JR, Miller DL, Nagorney DM et al (2001) Surgical treatment of hepatic and pulmonary metastases from colon cancer. Ann Thorac Surg 71:975-979
33. Kobayashi K, Kawamura M, Ishihara T (1999) Surgical treatment for both pulmonary and hepatic metastases from colorectal cancer. J Thorac Cardiovasc Surg 118:1090-1096
34. Shah SA, Haddad R, Al-Sukhni W et al (2006) Surgical resection of hepatic and pulmonary metastases from colorectal carcinoma. J Am Coll Surg 202:468-475
35. Nagakura S, Shirai Y, Yamato Y et al (2001) Simultaneous detection of colorectal carcinoma liver and lung metastases does not warrant resection. J Am Coll Surg 193:153-160
36. Mineo TC, Ambrogi V, Tonini G et al (2003) Longterm results after resection of simultaneous and sequential lung and liver metastases. J Am Coll Surg 197:386-391
37. Reddy RH, Kumar B, Shah R et al (2004) Staged pulmonary and hepatic metastasectomy in colorectal cancer - is it worth it? Eur J Cardiothorac Surg 25:151-154
38. Neeff H, Hörth W, Makowiec F et al (2009) Outcome after resection of hepatic and pulmonary metastases of colorectal cancer. J Gastrointest Surg. 13:1813-1820
39. Byam J, Reuter NP, Woodall CE et al (2009) Should hepatic metastatic colorectal cancer patients with extrahepatic disease undergo liver resection/ablation? Ann Surg Oncol 6:3064-3069
40. de Haas RJ, Rahy Martin AC, Wicherts DA et al (2009) Long-term outcome in patients with adrenal metastases following resection of colorectal liver metastases. Br J Surg 96:935-940

Adjuvant Chemotherapy and Follow-Up   10

Abstract Even though there are no definitive data supporting the use of adjuvant chemotherapy after liver resection for initially resectable hepatic colorectal metastases, the rationale for this approach seems evident. The activity of chemotherapy in metastatic disease is well known, and it is broadly accepted that, at least theoretically, patients with micrometastatic disease after radical surgery will benefit from systemic chemotherapy, as will patients undergoing surgery for stage III colon cancer.

10. 1
Introduction

Adjuvant chemotherapy is currently accepted as the standard approach following resection of node-positive primary colorectal cancers. Several trials have shown a significant survival benefit of adjuvant treatment with 5-fluoruracil (FU)-based chemotherapy over surgery alone [1-4]. The absolute benefit for adjuvant treatment appears to increase with the risk of relapse. In fact, whereas the benefit for node-positive (stage III) patients is quite clear, the role of adjuvant treatment for node-negative (stage II) patients is controversial [5, 6].

There are several options available for adjuvant chemotherapy in patients with stage III colon cancer. The current standard includes a combination of 6 months of infusional FU, folinic acid (LV), and oxaliplatin in the FOLFOX regimen, and the combination of 6 months oral capecitabine and infusional oxaliplatin in the XELOX regimen. Two pivotal studies (the MOSAIC trial [7] and the NSABP C-07 trial [8]) showed an improvement in 3-year disease-free survival—which has been widely accepted as a reliable surrogate end-point for overall survival [9]—in the oxaliplatin arm. More recently, in stage III patients, capecitabine, an oral prodrug of FU, was shown to be equally effective and better tolerated than monthly bolus FU [10, 11]. Finally, in a large study (the XELOXA trial), Haller et al. [12] demonstrated the statistically significant advantage of a combination of capecitabine and oxaliplatin over FU and LV infusional treatment, in terms of progression-free survival.

F. Leone (✉)
Division of Medical Oncology, Institute for Cancer Research and Treatment, Candiolo (TO), Italy

Surgical Treatment of Colorectal Liver Metastases. Lorenzo Capussotti (Ed.)   **153**
© Springer-Verlag Italia 2011

Given the high rate of recurrence after complete surgical resection of liver metastases, the use of adjuvant chemotherapy after hepatic resection appears rationale. Nonetheless, only a few clinical trials have specifically addressed the question of the impact of adjuvant chemotherapy on clinical outcomes, comparing systemic chemotherapy to observation after surgery.

10.2
Adjuvant Chemotherapy

In a large retrospective bi-institutional study of 792 liver resections (Memorial Sloan-Kettering Cancer Center, NY, USA and The Royal Infirmary of Edinburgh, Edinburgh, Scotland), 518 patients treated with surgery alone were compared with 274 patients treated with FU-based adjuvant chemotherapy following hepatic resection [13]. Patient survival was analyzed with stratification by a clinical risk score according to a previously described scoring system (see Chapter 5, "Results of Surgery and Prognostic Factors") [14]. The study found a statistically significant improvement of survival in patients who had received adjuvant chemotherapy; this was true even after stratification by clinical risk score. Adjuvant chemotherapy after hepatic resection for colorectal metastases was an independent predictor of outcome.

Several studies comparing adjuvant hepatic arterial infusion (HAI) chemotherapy with fluorodeoxyuridine (FUDR) to surgery alone demonstrated a significant increase in disease-free survival in the treated group. Overall survival was increased in two studies [15, 16], but the largest study, by Lorenz et al. [17] (226 patients), stopped after a planned interim analysis that showed HAI-related toxicity and intention-to-treat negative results for disease-free survival and overall survival. In a study in which patients were randomized to receive postoperative HAI in combination with systemic continuous FU or surgery alone, a significant improvement in 4-year recurrence rate (46% vs 25%) was demonstrated in patients receiving adjuvant therapy [18]. Two studies of combined HAI chemotherapy and intravenous systemic chemotherapy vs. intravenous chemotherapy alone showed an increase in disease-free survival in favor of combination therapy [19, 20]. In a similar design trial including 156 patients, Kemeny et al. [21] reported an increased overall survival in the combined treatment group after 2 years. Yet, the updated results after 5 years did not confirm the survival advantage [22]. In addition, HAI chemotherapy requires surgical implantation of a hepatic arterial catheter and the use of an implantable pump. Compliance with this treatment is therefore limited by a high rate of induced specific complications. For these reasons, although HAI chemotherapy has proved to reduce hepatic recurrences and increase survival, its application is greatly impaired by technical difficulties and case-specific complications.

More recently, in a multicenter phase III study, the FFCD trial [23], patients with completely resected (R0) hepatic metastases from colorectal cancer were randomized to surgery alone and observation or to surgery followed by 6 months of systemic adjuvant chemotherapy with FU and folinic acid. The primary end-point was disease-free survival. The study demonstrated that systemic chemotherapy provides a significant benefit over surgery alone. In the Cox multivariate analysis 5-year disease-free survival rate was 33.5% in the chemotherapy group vs. 26.7% in the control group. Although a trend towards increased overall survival was observed, it did not reach statistical significance. The ENG trial [24] produced similar results. Moreover, both studies closed prematurely because of slow accrual, thus lacking the statistical power to demonstrate the predefined difference in survival. However, a pooled analysis of these two studies showed a statistical significance in favor of adjuvant chemotherapy with a FU-based regimen (median overall survival was 62.2 months in the adjuvant-chemotherapy arm compared with 47.3 months in the surgery-alone arm) [25].

The most recent study on adjuvant chemotherapy following complete resection of liver metastases from colorectal cancer is a phase III multicenter study of 321 patients randomly assigned to receive either FU/LV or FOLFIRI as adjuvant chemotherapy [26]. The results of this trial evidenced no significant differences in overall survival between the two arms. In an unplanned exploratory analysis, in 158 patients who received treatment within a 6-week time-line following resection of liver metastases, those who received FOLFIRI had longer disease-free survival than patients receiving FU/LV, although this difference was not statistically significant.

While there is not yet clear evidence that combination therapies offer significant additional benefit to FU-based chemotherapy, nonetheless, combination chemotherapy with irinotecan or oxaliplatin is largely used in this setting. In general, it is believed that if colorectal cancer patients in stage III have a greater benefit from adjuvant oxaliplatin-based chemotherapy than from FU/LV, the same benefit should be maintained in stage IV resected patients. The safety and efficacy of combination chemotherapy in patients with metastatic disease are well documented, and the use of this approach in the treatment of micrometastatic disease seems to be rational. New clinical trials to investigate combinations of cytotoxic drugs and targeted agents are therefore encouraged. Considerations for tailoring combination therapy to include bevacizumab or the anti-EGFR monoclonal antibodies cetuximab and panitumumab in the adjuvant treatment after complete surgical resection will need to be addressed in future trials.

Despite the theoretical advantages of adjuvant chemotherapy, it must be kept in mind that long recovery times after extensive hepatic resections may result in chemotherapy starting too late to be of full benefit (when micrometastatic disease has already become established) and in poor tolerance of the adjuvant treatment [27].

10.3
Follow-Up

Recurrence rates after liver resection for colorectal cancer metastases are high. Nearly two-thirds of patients who undergo primary liver surgery for metastatic colorectal cancer experience tumor progression during further follow-up. Moreover, up to 90% of patients who are eligible for surgery after tumor downsizing by neoadjuvant chemotherapy are expected to develop a recurrence, usually soon after liver resection. Recurrences are frequently extrahepatic, either alone or associated with hepatic disease. Several studies demonstrated that re-resection, when feasible, is the preferred treatment for resectable recurrence [28-31] and that the most important independent predictor of improved disease-free survival is surgical resection of the recurrence. Also, extrahepatic disease should not be viewed as an absolute contraindication to resection because, in the case of limited disease involving one site, it can be considered as curative surgery.

Current level I evidence favors intensive surveillance programs after resection of a colorectal cancer. This recommendation is based on randomized trials [31, 32], meta-analyses [33, 34], and a systematic Cochrane review [35] showing a survival advantage in the group of patients followed more strictly. The benefit associated with a high-intensity follow-up program is explained by the earlier diagnosis of tumor recurrences, leading to higher rates of secondary curative intent surgery. Therefore, scientific societies, such as the American Society of Clinical Oncology, have proposed practice guideline for postoperative follow-up [36, 37]. However, neither studies nor definite guidelines are available to define the optimal follow-up scheme after radical resection of colorectal liver metastases. Yet, with the aim of detecting tumour recurrence potentially amenable to secondary resection, a close follow-up program is justified. Accordingly, it is important to monitor these patients regularly and more frequently in the first 3 years, when most recurrences occur. Most of the hepatobiliary centers employ a follow-up scheme consisting of clinical examination, serum carcinoembryonic antigen quantification, and liver ultrasound examination every 4 months together with a chest X-ray. Thoraco-abdominal computed tomography scan, performed at least yearly, is recommended as well.

References

1. International Multicentre Pooled Analysis of Colon Cancer Trials (IMPACT) investigators (1995) Efficacy of adjuvant fluorouracil and folinic acid in colon cancer. Lancet 345:939-944
2. Goldberg RM, Hatfield AK, Kahn M et al (1997) Prospectively randomized North Central Cancer Treatment Group trial of intensive-course fluorouracil combined with the l-isomer of intravenous leucovorin, oral leucovorin, or intravenous leucovorin for the treatment of advanced colorectal cancer. J Clin Oncol 15:3320-3329
3. Moertel CG, Fleming TR, Macdonald JS et al (1995) Fluorouracil plus levamisole as effective adjuvant therapy after resection of stage III colon carcinoma: a final report. Ann Intern Med 122:321-326
4. Wolmark N, Rockette H, Fisher B et al (1993) The benefit of leucovorin-modulated fluorouracil as postoperative adjuvant therapy for primary colon cancer: results from National Surgical Adjuvant Breast and Bowel Project protocol C-03. J Clin Oncol 11:1879-1887
5. Mamounas E, Wieand S, Wolmark N et al (1999) Comparative efficacy of adjuvant chemotherapy in patients with Dukes' B versus Dukes' C colon cancer: results from four National Surgical Adjuvant Breast and Bowel Project adjuvant studies (C-01, C-02, C-03, and C-04). J Clin Oncol 17:1349-55

6. Efficacy of adjuvant fluorouracil and folinic acid in B2 colon cancer. International Multicentre Pooled Analysis of B2 Colon Cancer Trials (IMPACT B2) Investigators. (1999) J Clin Oncol 17:1356-63

7. Andre T, Boni C, Mounedji-Boudiaf L et al (2004) Oxaliplatin, fluorouracil, and leucovorin as adjuvant treatment for colon cancer. N Engl J Med 350:2343-2351

8. Wolmark N, Kuebler JP, Colangelo L et al (2005) A phase III trial comparing FULV to FULV + oxaliplatin in stage II or III carcinoma of the colon: Results of NSABP Protocol C-07. Proc Amer Soc Clin Oncol (abstr # 3500)

9. Sargent DJ, Wieand HS, Haller DG et al (2005) Disease-free survival versus overall survival as a primary end point for adjuvant colon cancer studies: individual patient data from 20,898 patients on 18 randomized trials. J Clin Oncol 23:8664-8670

10. Twelves C, Wong A, Nowacki MP et al (2005) Capecitabine as adjuvant treatment for stage III colon cancer (X-ACT Trial). N Engl J Med 352:2696-2704

11. Scheithauer W, McKendrick J, Begbie et al (2003) Oral capecitabine as an alternative to i.v. 5-fluorouracil-based adjuvant therapy for colon cancer: Safety results of a randomized, phase III trial. Ann Oncol 14:1735-1743

12. Haller D, Tabernero J, Maroun J et al (2009) First efficacy findings from a randomized phase III trial of capecitabine + oxaliplatin vs. bolus 5-FU/LV for stage III colon cancer (NO16968/XELOXA study). Joint ECCO 15 – 34th ESMO Multidisciplinary Congress. Abstract #5LBA

13. Parks R, Gonen M, Kemeny N et al (2007) Adjuvant chemotherapy improves survival after resection of hepatic colorectal metastases: analysis of data from two continents. J Am Coll Surg 204:753-761

14. Fong Y, Fortner JG, Sun R et al (1999) Clinical score for predicting recurrence after hepatic resection for metastatic colorectal cancer: analysis of 1001 consecutive cases. Ann Surg 230:309–321

15. Lygidakis NJ, Ziras N, Parissis J (1995) Resection versus resection combined with adjuvant pre- and post-operative chemotherapy–immunotherapy for metastatic colorectal liver cancer. A new look at an old problem. Hepatogastroenterology 42:155-161

16. Asahara T, Kikkawa M, Okajima M et al (1998) Studies of postoperative transarterial infusion chemotherapy for liver metastasis of colorectal carcinoma after hepatectomy. Hepatogastroenterology 45:805-811

17. Lorenz M, Müller HH, Schramm H et al (1998) Randomized trial of surgery versus surgery followed by adjuvant hepatic arterial infusion with 5-fluorouracil and folinic acid for liver metastases of colorectal cancer: German Cooperative on Liver Metastases (Arbeitsgruppe Lebermetastasen). Ann Surg 228:756-762

18. Kemeny MM, Adak S, Gray B et al (2002) Combined-modality treatment for resectable metastatic colorectal carcinoma to the liver: Surgical resection of hepatic metastases in combination with continuous infusion of chemotherapy–an Intergroup study. J Clin Oncol 20:1499-1505

19. Tono T, Hasuike Y, Ohzato H et al (2000) Limited but definite efficacy of prophylactic hepatic arterial infusion chemotherapy after curative resection of colorectal liver metastases: A randomized study. Cancer 88:1549-1556

20. Lygidakis NJ, Sgourakis G, Vlachos L et al (2001) Metastatic liver disease of colorectal origin: The value of locoregional immunochemotherapy combined with systemic chemotherapy following liver resection: Results of a prospective randomized study. Hepatogastroenterology 48:1685-1691

21. Kemeny N, Huang Y, Cohen AM et al (1999) Hepatic arterial infusion of chemotherapy after resection of hepatic metastases from colorectal cancer. N Engl J Med 341:2039-2048

22. Kemeny NE, Gonen M (2005) Hepatic arterial infusion after liver resection. N Engl J Med 352:734-735

23. Portier G, Elias D, Bouche O et al (2006) Multicenter randomized trial of adjuvant fluorouracil and folinic acid compared with surgery alone after resection of colorectal liver metastases: FFCD ACHBTH AURC 9002 trial. J Clin Oncol 24:4976–4982
24. Langer B, Bleiberg H, Labianca R et al (2002) Fluorouracil (FU) plus l-leucovorin (l-LV) versus observation after potentially curative resection of liver or lung metastases from colorectal cancer (CRC): Results of the ENG (EORTC/NCIC CTG/GIVIO) randomized trial. J Clin Oncol 21(abstr 592)
25. Mitry E, Fields A, Bleiberg H et al (2008) Adjuvant chemotherapy after potentially curative resection of metastases from colorectal cancer. A meta-analysis of two randomized trials. J Clin Oncol 26:4906–4911
26. Ychou1 M, Hohenberger W, Thezenas S et al (2009) A randomized phase III study comparing adjuvant 5-fluorouracil/folinic acid with FOLFIRI in patients following complete resection of liver metastases from colorectal cancer. Ann Oncol 20:1964–1970
27. Power DG, Kemeny NE (2010) Role of adjuvant therapy after resection of colorectal cancer liver metastases. J Clin Oncol 28:2300-2309
28. Muratore A, Polastri R, Bouzari H et al (2001) Repeat hepatectomy for colorectal liver metastases: a worthwhile operation? J Surg Oncol 76:127–132
29. Petrowsky H, Gonen M, Jarnagin W et al (2002) Second liver resections are safe and effective treatment for recurrent hepatic metastases from colorectal cancer: a bi-institutional analysis. Ann Surg 235:863–871
30. Adam R, Pascal G, Azoulay D et al (2003) Liver resection for colorectal metastases: the third hepatectomy. Ann Surg 238:871–884
31. Saito Y, Omiya H, Kohno K et al (2002) Pulmonary metastasectomy for 165 patients with colorectal carcinoma: a prognostic assessment. J Thorac Cardiovasc Surg 124:1007–1013
32. Secco GB, Fardelli R, Gianquinto D et al (2002) Efficacy and cost of risk adapted follow-up in patients after colorectal cancer surgery: a prospective, randomized and controlled trial. Eur J Surg Oncol 28:418–423
33. Rodriguez-Moranta F, Salo J, Arcusa A et al (2005) Postoperative surveillance in patients with colorectal cancer who have undergone curative resection: A prospective, multicenter, randomized, controlled trial. J Clin Oncol 24:1–8
34. Figueredo A, Rumble RB, Maroun J et al (2003) Gastrointestinal Cancer Disease Site Group of Cancer Care Ontario's. Follow-up of patients with curatively resected colorectal cancer: a practice guideline. BMC Cancer 3:26
35. Tjandra JJ, Chan MK (2007) Follow-up after curative resection of colorectal cancer: a meta-analysis. Dis Col Rect 50:1783-1799
36. Desch CE, Benson III AB, Somerfield MR et al (2005) Colorectal Cancer Surveillance: 2005 Update of an American Society of Clinical Oncology Practice Guideline. J Clin Oncol 23:8512-8519
37. Tsikitis VL, Malireddy K, Green EA et al (2009) Postoperative surveillance recommendations for early stage colon cancer based on results from the clinical outcomes of surgical therapy trial. J Clin Oncol 27:3671-3676

Re-resection: Indications and Results 11

Abstract Intrahepatic recurrence after curative liver resection is a common event. In the last 15 years, the rate of re-resection of a liver recurrence has progressively increased such that up to 20% of patients with an intrahepatic recurrence are now expected to undergo re-resection. Although re-resection is technically more demanding, mortality/morbidity and long-term survival rates are similar to those reported for initial liver resection. The major indication for re-resection is the technical feasibility of a curative procedure.

11.1
Introduction

Advances in surgical and medical oncology have resulted in the prolongation of survival for patients with colorectal metastases who have undergone curative resection; however, many patients will still develop disease recurrence [1]. A recent paper analyzed the recurrence pattern in 1669 patients who had curative liver surgery for colorectal metastases at four major hepatobiliary centers in the USA (John Hopkins School of Medicine, Baltimore, MD) and Europe (Hopitaux Universitaries de Geneve, Geneva, Switzerland; Ospedale San Raffaele, Milan, Italy, Ospedale Mauriziano "Umberto I", Turin, Italy). Of the 947 patients (57.7%) who developed a recurrence, the disease was intrahepatic only in 409 patients (43.2%), intra- and extrahepatic in 199 (21%), and extrahepatic only in 339 (35.8%) [2]. Overall, two thirds of the recurrences were intrahepatic, with a median time to recurrence of 17 months.

Thus, although liver recurrence is a common event after curative resection of colorectal liver metastases, until the 1990s a liver recurrence was an uncommon indication for re-resection, with few anecdotal cases reported by the major hepatobiliary centers. Nonetheless, it was already well-accepted that surgical excision of a localized liver recurrence could be an effective treatment, with long-term outcomes that did not differ greatly from those associated with the initial resection [3, 4]. The early 1990s had seen the publication of two large series of repeat liver resections for

---

A. Muratore (✉)
Division of Hepato-Bilio-Pancreatic and Digestive Surgery, Mauriziano "Umberto I" Hospital,
Turin, Italy

Surgical Treatment of Colorectal Liver Metastases. Lorenzo Capussotti (Ed.) **159**
© Springer-Verlag Italia 2011

colorectal metastases: overall, 300 patients received 321 repeat liver resections with a 3-year survival ranging from 33% to 45% [5, 6]. In the following years, the number of publications reporting re-resection of colorectal liver metastases progressively increased, and a Medline search currently lists more than 100 papers on this procedure and its results.

11.2
Short-term Outcome

Nowadays, up to 20% of the patients with a liver recurrence are expected to undergo re-resection [7, 8]. In our series (from January 1989 to December 2009), 125 of 668 patients (18.7%) treated by resection underwent re-resection for a liver recurrence: 2nd liver resection in 125 patients, 3rd liver resection in 18, and 4th liver resection in 1. Repeat hepatectomies are more difficult than initial resections for several reasons. Firstly, regeneration of the liver induces modifications of its shape and of the disposition of its vascular structures, making pre- and intraoperative resection planning more complex. Secondly, re-exposure of the hepatic pedicle and of the portion of the liver to be resected is more difficult due to the presence of adhesions of the liver surface to either adjacent organs or the diaphragm. Thirdly, the liver parenchyma is often more fragile as a consequence of regeneration and preoperative chemotherapy. However, despite the often increased operative time of repeat colorectal liver resection, compared with the initial liver resection, in-hospital mortality and morbidity rates are the same [9] and currently range from 0% to 1.6% and from 18% to 28%, respectively (Table 11.1). Similarly, no significant differences have been observed in perioperative blood loss and length of hospital stay after repeat hepatic resection. A multicenter study found that up to two-thirds of the patients had a blood loss of < 100 ml and the mean hospital stay was 9 days [9]. However, it must be kept in mind that these excellent results are reported from specialized hepatobiliary centers.

The extent of hepatic resection obviously decreases with repeat hepatic resection (≥ 4 segments: 30.9% after 1st hepatic resection, 21.1% after 2nd hepatic resection, 16.4% after 3rd–4th hepatic resection) [9].

Table 11.1 Morbidity and mortality rates after repeat hepatic resection

Authors	Year	Patients (*n*)	Mortality (%)	Morbidity (%)
Petrowski [8]	2002	126	1.6	28
Adam[a] [10]	2003	60	0	25
Shaw [11]	2006	66	0	18
de Jong [9]	2009	246	0.4	22.5
Brachet [12]	2009	62	0	20

[a]Third hepatectomy

11.3
Long-term Outcome

Repeat hepatic resections are also technically more demanding and difficult, but they are safe in terms of curative resection compared with the initial hepatectomy. Indeed, the same multicenter study cited above found significantly better radical (R0) resection rates after repeat hepatic resection: with a rate of 90.2% after repeat hepatic resection vs. 79.8% after 1st hepatic resection ($p = 0.01$) [9]. One possible explanation is patient selection, as significantly lower rates of multiple, bilateral metastases are reported among patients undergoing repeat hepatectomies than in those receiving their first hepatectomy [8, 9]. However, the overall rate of R0 resection reported in the literature is high (80–90%) [7, 10]. By contrast, in our series, the rate of R0 resection was not significantly different between 1st and 2nd liver resections (83% vs. 93%, respectively).

The benefit provided by 2nd hepatic resection is evidenced by the 5-year survival rates, which range from 22% to 44% [6, 8, 9, 12, 13] (Table 11.2). Furthermore, patients undergoing a third hepatic resection show similar 5-year survival rates: 24–32% from the time of the third hepatic resection and 65–78% from the time of the first hepatic resection [9, 10]. Obviously, as with first hepatic resection, in repeat resection the issue of appropriate patient selection, i.e., those with a more favorable prognosis, is also important.

Many studies have analyzed the prognostic factors correlated with a better long-term outcome after repeat hepatic resection, but the results are conflicting (Table 11.3). Nonetheless, patients with negative prognostic factors, such as large, multiple metastases or the presence of extrahepatic disease, still have significantly better 3-year survival rates (around 30%) than the 5% reported for patients ineligible for liver resection [8, 10]. The most common and important prognostic factor of survival seems to be the curative pattern of the repeat hepatic resection. The presence of residual disease (especially if extrahepatic) at the end of the repeat hepatic resection is an independent prognostic factor of worse survival in most of the reported series

Table 11.2 Three- and five- year survival rates after repeat hepatic resection

Authors	Year	Patients (*n*)	3-year survival (%)	5-year survival (%)
Adam [13]	1997	64	60	41
Imamura [14]	2000	20	59	22
Petrowski [8]	2002	126	51	34
Shaw [11]	2006	66	68	44
de Jong [9]	2009	246	–	32.6
Brachet [12]	2009	62	–	40

Table 11.3 Predictors of outcome after repeat hepatic resection

Author	Year	Patients (*n*)	Prognostic factors
Fernandez-Trigo [6]	1995	170	R0/+ resection
Adam [13]	1997	64	Interval 1st–2nd hepatectomy (1 vs. > 1 year) R0/+ resection
Petrowski [8]	2002	126	Tumor number (single vs. multiple) Tumor size (<5 vs. ≥ 3 cm)
Adam[a] [10]	2003	60	Tumor size at 1st resection (≤ 3 vs. > 3 cm) Extrahepatic disease R0/+ resection
de Jong [9]	2009	246	Extrahepatic disease
Brachet [12]	2009	62	CEA serum level at 1st liver resection Anatomic resection Tumor size (< 3 vs. ≥3 cm)

[a]Third hepatectomy

[6, 10, 13]. Therefore, it is now agreed that the indications for repeat hepatic resection should be the same as those for the first hepatic resection, i.e., surgery is indicated whenever colorectal liver metastases are technically resectable in terms of curative effect, regardless of disease extent.

In conclusion, about 20% of the patients who develop a liver recurrence after curative resection of colorectal liver metastases will undergo re-resection of the recurrence. Despite the fact that repeat hepatic resections are technically more demanding, reports of series from specialized hepatobiliary centers have demonstrated morbidity/mortally and curative resection rates similar to those obtained with the initial liver resection. The long-term survival benefit of repeat hepatic resections is therefore beyond any doubt, provided that the liver resection is technically feasible and curative.

References

1. Capussotti L, Muratore A, Mulas M et al (2006) Neoadjuvant chemotherapy and resection for initially irresectable colorectal liver metastases. Br J Surg 93:1001-1006
2. de Jong MC, Pulitano C, Ribero D et al (2009) Rates and patterns of recurrence following curative intent surgery for colorectal liver metastasis. An international multi-institutional analysis of 1669 patients. Ann Surg 250:440-448
3. Huguet C, Boba S, Nordlinger B et al (1990) Repaet hepatic resection for primary and metastatic carcinoma of the liver. Surgery Gynecol & Obstetrics 171:398-402

4. Fortner JG. (1988) Recurrence of colorectal cancer after hepatic resection. Am J Surg 155:378-382
5. Nordlinger B, Vaillant JC, Guiguet M et al (1994) Survival benefit of repeat liver resections for recurrent colorectal metastases: 143 cases. J Clin Oncol 12:1491-1496
6. Fernandez-Trigo V, Shamsa F et al (1995) Repeat liver resection for colorectal metastasis. Surgery 117:296-304
7. Muratore A, Polastri R, Bouzari H et al (2001) Repeat hepatectomy for colorectal liver metastases: a worthwhile operation? J Surg Oncol 76:127-132
8. Petrowsky H, Gonen M, Jarnagin W et al (2002) Second liver resections are safe and effective treatment for recurrent hepatic metastases from colorectal cancer. A bi-institutional analysis. Ann Surg 235:863-871
9. de Jong M, Mayo SC, Pulitano C et al (2009) Repeat curative intent liver surgery is safe and effective for recurrent colorectal liver metastasis: results from an international multi-institutional analysis. J Gastroint Surg 13:2141-2151
10. Adam R, Pascal G, Azoulay D et al (2003) Liver resection for colorectal metastases. The third hepatectomy. Ann Surg 238:871-884
11. Shaw MI, Rees M, Welsh FKS et al (2006) Repeat hepatic resection for recurrent colorectal liver metastases is associated with favourable long-term survival. Br J Surg 93:457-464
12. Brachet D, Dermite E, Rouquette A et al (2009) Prognostic factors of survival in repeat liver resection for recurrent colorectal metastases: review of sixty-two cases treated at a single institution. Dis Colon Rectum 52:475-483
13. Adam R, Bismuth H, Castaing D et al (1997) Repeat hepatectomy for colorectal liver metastases. Ann Surg 225:51-62
14. Imamura H, Kawasaki S, Miyagawa S et al (2000) Aggressive surgical approach to recurrent tumours after hepatectomy for metastatic spread of colorectal cancer to the liver. Surgery 127:528-535

LiverMetSurvey Registry: the Italian Experience

12

Abstract LiverMetSurvey (www.livermetsurvey.org) is an international registry of patients who have undergone surgery for colorectal liver metastases. It aims to analyze prospectively, on a large scale, the results of surgically treated patients, with the broader goal of establishing guidelines of optimal treatment and therapeutic strategy, especially in clinical situations that remain controversial regarding the benefit of surgery or its combination with other therapies. All patients who have undergone resection of hepatic metastasis of colorectal origin, whether the hepatectomy was actually performed or canceled during the operation (intention-to-treat), are included. As of December 2009, more than 11,000 patients have been registered worldwide. In this chapter, data from Italian centers participating in LiverMetSurvey are analyzed in order to illustrate the outcomes of surgical treatment of colorectal liver metastases in our country. Furthermore, the Italian data are compared with those of the LiverMetSurvey series such that treatment quality in Italy can be compared to international standards.

12.1
Introduction

LiverMetSurvey (www.livermetsurvey.org) is an international registry of patients who have undergone surgery for colorectal liver metastases. It was founded in 2004 by Prof. René Adam and Prof. Gérard Pascal of the Paul Brousse Hospital (Villejuif, France) together with an international scientific board of hepatobiliary experts (Arvidsson D, Stockholm, Sweden; Bechstein W, Frankfurt, Germany; Barroso E, Lisbon, Portugal; Capussotti L, Torino, Italy; Clavien PA, Zurich, Switzerland; Figueras J, Barcelona, Spain; Garden J, Edinburgh, UK; Gigot JF, Brussels, Belgium; Jaeck D, Strasbourg, France; Mentha G, Geneva, Switzerland; Poston G, Liverpool, UK; Verhoef C, Rotterdam, Netherlands). The LiverMetSurvey is a descriptive, observational, retrospective and prospective, multicenter, international study focused on surgical fields involved in the care of patients with hepatic metastases.

L. Viganò (✉)
Division of Hepato-Bilio-Pancreatic and Digestive Surgery, Mauriziano "Umberto I" Hospital, Turin, Italy

Surgical Treatment of Colorectal Liver Metastases. Lorenzo Capussotti (Ed.)
© Springer-Verlag Italia 2011

It comprises all patients of each center who underwent surgery for hepatic metastases of colorectal origin. All patients who underwent surgery for resection of hepatic metastasis of colorectal origin, whether the hepatectomy was performed or canceled during the operation, are included (intention-to-treat).

The objectives of the registry are:

- To collect and analyze, on an international multi-institutional basis, critical data of patients surgically treated for hepatic metastases of colorectal origin.
- To describe this population, the therapeutic procedures, and the outcomes.
- To analyze the results (survival, recurrence) of the treatments (resection, adjuvant treatment, chemotherapy).
- To compare the outcome of patients with respect to characteristics at inclusion and to therapeutic procedures, thereby identifying potential prognostic factors.

The LiverMetSurvey registry aims to prospectively analyze, on a large scale, the results of surgically treated patients, with the broader goal of establishing guidelines of optimal treatment and therapeutic strategy, especially in clinical situations that remain controversial with respect to the benefit of surgery or its adequate combination with other therapies.

The LiverMetSurvey registry is open to all centers throughout the world. Any hospital center performing liver surgery can participate; there are no selection criteria related to prior surgical experience or to the size of the center.

The prospective online inclusion of patient data started in January 2005; however, participating centers were allowed to register data describing their entire series of patients who underwent resection before January 2005, provided that the information had been prospectively collected, that it could be entered in the format of the questionnaire, and that the quality of the data could be properly assessed by the data manager. Participation in the study requires mandatory participation in the prospective arm of the study whereas participation in the retrospective arm is optional.

The registry is set up within a center through an online Internet application. This method ensures the quality of the data through online data entry assistance and controls. Data are entered in the registry using a standardized questionnaire that was formulated by the scientific committee. The following information must be entered:

- Patient characteristics (sex, date, and place of birth).
- Primary colorectal cancer (location, TNM staging) and treatment (surgery, chemotherapy) description.
- Hepatic metastasis description (occurrence date, number, size, location, resectability, treatment).
- Extrahepatic metastasis description (location, treatment).
- Treatment description:
  - pre- and post-surgery chemotherapy (drugs, cycles, results);
  - hepatectomy characteristics (type, involved segments, vascular occlusion, laparoscopy, intraoperative ultrasonography, liver curative, globally curative);
  - surgery techniques aimed at allowing resection: portal embolization, combined treatments (cryotherapy, radiofrequency ablation), two-stage hepatectomy;
- Postoperative outcomes (mortality, morbidities, re-intervention, hospital stay).
- Histological findings (pathologic tumor characteristics, histology of non-tumoral liver).

- Recurrences characteristics:
  - hepatic recurrences (occurrence date, number, size, location, resectability, treatment):
  - extrahepatic recurrences (location, occurrence date, treatment);
- Updated patient information (alive/deceased, with/without recurrence).

Data are entered initially at the time of the surgery for hepatic metastasis, then during follow-up, and, optimally, each time new information is available or at least once a year. Each center updates its follow-up data on line, with a global review by the data manager every 6 months.

In this chapter, data from Italian centers participating in the LiverMetSurvey are analyzed in order to describe the outcomes of surgical treatment of colorectal liver metastases in our country. In addition, Italian data are compared with those of the entire LiverMetSurvey series, thus allowing treatment quality in Italy to be compared to international standards.

12.2
The Italian Experience

As of December 2009, 11,644 patients were registered in the LiverMetSurvey database from 180 centers of 56 different countries (Fig. 12.1). Of these, 10,722 patients underwent 12,457 liver resections. Italy has the largest number of participating centers (37) and, after France, has the highest number of included patients: 1827 (15.7%) patients, including 1709 (15.9%) undergoing liver resections. Ten centers have registered more than 50 patients. The distribution of centers in the different regions of Italy is shown in Fig. 12.2. Since 2005, the number of registered centers has increased every year, as has the number of included patients (Fig. 12.3). At present, more than 300 patients per year are enrolled in the LiverMetSurvey registry by Italian centers.

12.2.1
Patient Characteristics

The characteristics of the 1709 resected patients included in the LiverMetSurvey registry by Italian centers are summarized in Table 12.1. The number of patients for whom data are available is detailed in parentheses. There were 1045 males and 664 females; 413 (/1696, 24.4%) patients were over 70 years and 42 (2.5%) over 80. Primary rectal cancer was diagnosed in 463 patients (/1460, 31.7%). Colorectal cancer was stage T3 in 951 patients (/1330, 71.5%), T4 in 223 (16.8%), and N positive in 882 (/1318, 66.9%). Liver metastases were synchronous to the primary tumor in 726 patients (/1381, 52.6%) and bilobar in 432 (/1378, 31.6%). Liver deposits were multiple in 659 patients (/1301, 50.7%), > 3 in 237 (18.2%), and > 10 in 23 (1.8%). Metastases diameter was > 5 cm in 333 patients (/1225, 27.2%) and > 10 cm in 36 (2.9%).

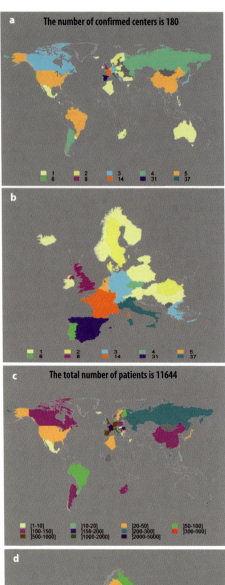
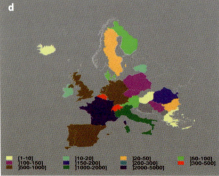

Fig. 12.1 Number of confirmed centers participating in the LiverMetSurvey registry and of included patients until December 2009. Number of confirmed centers per country in the world (**a**) and in Europe (**b**). Number of patients per country in the world (**c**) and in Europe (**d**)

12 LiverMetSurvey Registry: The Italian Experience

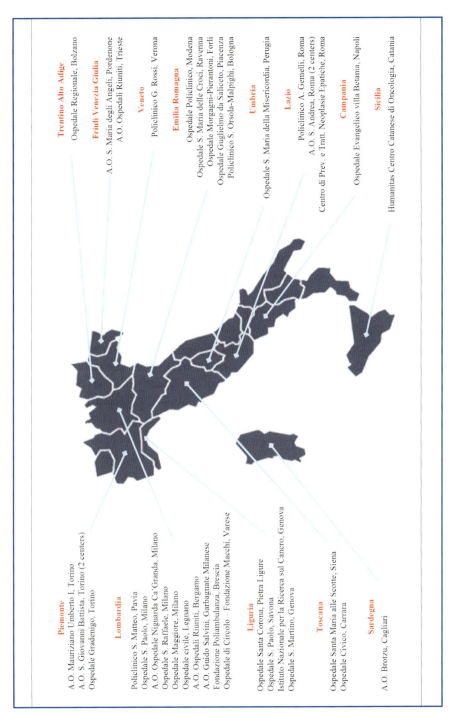

Fig. 12.2 Italian centers participating in the LiverMetSurvey registry

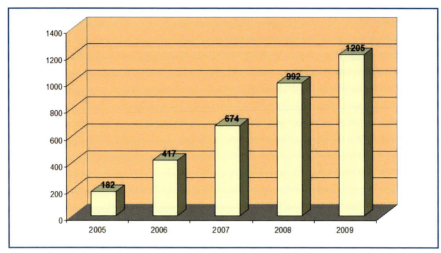

Fig. 12.3 Cumulative number of patients included in the prospective arm (since January 2005) of LiverMetSurvey by Italian centers

Table 12.1 Patient characteristics

Characteristic		n = 1709
Sex	Male	1045 (61.2%)
	Female	664 (38.8%)
Age	< 70	1272 (75.5%)
	70–75	241 (14.3%)
	75–80	130 (7.7%)
	≥ 80	42 (2.5%)
Primary colorectal cancer		
Tumor localization	Right	327 (22.4%)
	Transverse	56 (3.8%)
	Left/Sigmoid	585 (40.1%)
	Rectum	431 (29.5%)
	Multiple	61 (4.2%)
T stage	T0	5 (0.4%)
	T1	23 (1.7%)
	T2	128 (9.6%)
	T3	951 (71.5%)
	T4	223 (16.8%)
N Stage	N0	436 (33.1%)
	N1	535 (40.6%)
	N2	347 (26.3%)
Liver metastases		
Number	1–3	1064 (81.8%)
	> 3	237 (18.2%)
	> 5	120 (9.2%)
	> 10	23 (1.8%)

(Cont. →)

12 LiverMetSurvey Registry: The Italian Experience

Table 12.1 (continued)

Characteristic		n = 1709
Size	0–30 mm	636 (51.9%)
	30–50 mm	325 (26.5%)
	50–100 mm	228 (18.6%)
	> 100 mm	36 (2.9%)
Bilobar	Y	432 (31.4%)
	N	946 (68.7%)
Synchronous	Y	726 (52.6%)
	N	655 (47.4%)
Major hepatectomy	Y	831 (51.7%)
	N	775 (48.3%)
Radical resection	Y	1079 (81.3%)
	N	248 (18.7%)
Extrahepatic disease	Y	190 (11.1%)
	N	1518 (88.9%)

Slightly more than half of the patients (831/1606, 51.7%) underwent major liver resection. In the 190 (/1708, 11.1%) patients who had concomitant extrahepatic disease, the site distribution was as follows: lung in 54 (28.4%) patients, lymph nodes in 14 (7.4%), peritoneum in 9 (4.7%), multiple sites in 75 (39.5%), and other sites in 38 (20%). Resection was radical in 1079 patients (/1327, 81.3%).

Preoperative chemotherapy was administered to 598 patients (/1324, 45.2%), with FOLFOX as the commonest regimen (222 patients, 37.1%). Multiple chemotherapy lines were administered to 103 patients (/598, 17.2%). The number of chemotherapy cycles was > 6 in 262 patients (/501, 52.3%). Chemotherapy details are summarized in Table 12.2. Response to the last chemotherapy line was as follows: complete response in 32 patients (/543, 5.9%), partial response in 362 (66.7%), stable disease in 93 (17.1%), and disease progression in 56 (10.3%).

12.2.2
Short-term Outcomes

The 90-day mortality rate was 1.3%, with half of the deaths occurring within the first 30 postoperative days. Postoperative recovery was uneventful in 74% of the patients (880/1189), while morbidity occurred in 26%. Complications were classified as "hepatic" in 93 patients (/1189, 7.8%), "general" in 184 (15.5%), and "hepatic and general" in 32 (2.7%).

Table 12.2 Chemotherapy characteristics

		$n = 598$
Number of CTx lines	1	495 (82.8%)
	2	79 (13.2%)
	3	13 (2.2%)
	> 3	11 (1.8%)
Number of CTx cycles	1-6	239 (47.7%)
	7–12	203 (40.5%)
	13–18	36 (7.2%)
	19–24	16 (3.2%)
	> 24	7 (1.4%)
Last CTx line	5-FU	21 (3.5%)
	5-FU + Bevacizumab	5 (0.8%)
	Oxaliplatin	222 (37.1%)
	Oxaliplatin + Bevacizumab	25 (4.2%)
	Oxaliplatin + Cetuximab	3 (0.5%)
	Irinotecan	44 (7.4%)
	Irinotecan + Bevacizumab	70 (11.7%)
	Irinotecan + Cetuximab	6 (1.0%)
	Oxaliplatin + Irinotecan	21 (3.5%)
	Oxaliplatin + Irinotecan + Cetuximab	2 (0.3%)
	Other regimen	123 (20.6%)
	Unknown	56 (9.4%)
Response to the last CTx regimen	Complete Response	32 (5.9%)
	Partial Response	362 (66.7%)
	Stable Disease	93 (17.1%)
	Progression of Disease	56 (10.3%)

CTx, chemotherapy

12.2.3
Long-term Outcomes

Survival data are available for 1688 patients (/1709, 98.8%). After a median follow-up of 23.0 months, the 3- and 5-year survival rates of patients who underwent resection were 60% and 39%, respectively. In the present series, there are 154 5-year survivors and 34 10-year ones. The survival of patients who underwent resection was significantly higher than that of patients undergoing explorative laparotomy (3- and 5-year survival rates: 17% and 10% respectively, $p < 0.0001$; Fig. 12.4). There were only two 5-year survivors in the non-resected group.

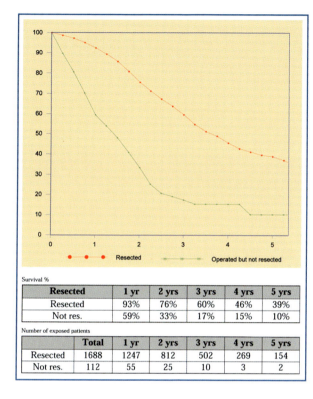

Fig. 12.4 Overall survival of patients who underwent resection vs. those who underwent surgery but not resection ($p < 0.0001$)

At last follow-up, 1055 out of 1688 patients were alive (62.5%); their status was disease-free in 674 (39.9%), with recurrence in 307 (18.2%), and unknown in 74 (4.4%). Among the remaining 633 patients (37.5%), 377 died because of disease progression (22.3%), 41 from non-tumoral causes (2.4%), and 215 from unknown causes (12.7%).

Recurrence site was documented in 366 patients and was classified as hepatic in 148 (40.4%), extrahepatic in 124 (33.9 %), and both in 94 (25.7%).

Among the 198 patients (/1709, 11.6%) who had liver re-resection, 17 (1.0%) required a third hepatectomy and one patient (0.1%) a fourth one. The survival rate of patients undergoing a second hepatectomy was 52% at 5 years from the first liver resection and 34% from the second one. This last result is similar to that of the whole series after the first hepatectomy (39%) (Fig. 12.5).

12.2.4
Prognostic Factors

The prognostic factors for overall survival are shown in Table 12.3. Demographic data and primary tumor localization had no impact on prognosis, in contrast to N stage of the primary tumor, which had a significant prognostic role (5-year survival rate 53% in N0 patients, 38% in N1, and 35% in N2, $p < 0.0001$). Many characteristics

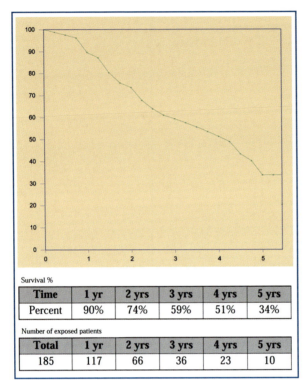

Fig. 12.5 Overall survival of patients after second hepatectomy for recurrent liver metastases

Table 12.3 Univariate analysis of prognostic factors of overall survival

		#	Survival (%) 1-year	3-year	5-year	Univariate p
Sex	M	1028	93	61	38	n.s.
	F	660	92	58	40	
Age (years)	< 70	1272	93	59	39	n.s.
	≥ 70	408	90	61	39	
Tumor localization	Right	320	90	55	37	n.s.
	Transverse	56	96	71	52	
	Left/Sigmoid	577	94	63	43	
	Rectum	428	93	61	37	
	Multiple	60	84	57	29	
T stage	T0	5	100			n.s.
	T1	23	100	77	48	
	T2	124	96	65	47	
	T3	940	93	64	44	
	T4	222	91	53	32	

(*Cont.* →)

Table 12.3 (continued)

		#	Survival (%)			Univariate
			1-year	3-year	5-year	p
N stage	N0	431	97	72	53	< 0.0001
	N1	529	92	61	38	
	N2	343	89	44	35	
Metastases number	1-3	1049	94	67	49	< 0.0001
	>3	235	88	42	14	
Metastases size (mm)	< 50	880	93	63	44	0.003
	≥ 50	330	91	52	30	
Metastases localization	Bilobar	426	91	54	31	0.0002
	Unilobar	933	93	65	47	
Synchronous	Y	717	92	59	39	n.s.
	N	645	92	64	45	
Major hepatectomy	Y	822	91	56	34	0.01
	N	765	94	61	44	
Extrahepatic disease	Y	188	89	42	17	< 0.0001
	N	1499	93	62	41	
Radical resection	Y	1062	93	66	48	< 0.0001
	N	247	89	45	22	
Initial resectability	Y	1122	93	64	45	0.0002
	N	207	90	47	20	
Preoperative CTx	Y	596	93	58	35	n.s.
	N	709	92	64	48	
Number of CTx lines	1	493	93	58	38	n.s.
	2	79	91	62	30	
	3	13	100	39	26	
	>3	11	100	69		
Number of CTx cycles	1-6	237	94	57	44	n.s.
	> 6	261	93	63	36	
Response to the last	CR	32	96	83	83	0.024
CTx regimen	PR	361	95	61	40	
	SD	93	92	58	34	
	PD	56	89	48	14	

CR, complete response; *CTx*, chemotherapy; *PD*, progression of disease; *PR*, partial response; *SD*, stable disease of the metastases were related to survival. First, the number of lesions: patients with more than three metastases had significantly lower survival rates (at 5 years 14% vs. 49%, $p < 0.0001$; Fig. 12.6a), increasing the number of nodules prognosis did not further worsen. Second, tumor size: patients with lesions > 50 mm had poorer outcomes (5-year survival rate 30% vs. 44%, $p = 0.003$; Fig. 12.6b), and survival further decreased in patients with metastases > 100 mm (at 5 years: 19%), but the difference was not statistically significant. Patients with synchronous liver metastases did not have a worse prognosis than those with metachronous ones. Further prognostic factors were bilateral localization of metastases (5 years: 31% vs. 47%, $p = 0.0002$), the need for major hepatectomy (34% vs. 44%, $p = 0.01$), and concomitant extrahepatic disease (17% vs. 41%, $p < 0.0001$).

As expected, R0 resection corresponded to better survival outcomes. The 5-year survival rate for these patients was 48% after complete resection vs. 22% after a non-radical one, $p < 0.0001$ (Fig. 12.7). Of note, only six out of 247 (2.4%) patients who received a non-radical resection were alive 5 years after the procedure.

Considering chemotherapy, preoperative treatment did not correspond to survival improvement. However, the two groups were not comparable because patients receiving preoperative chemotherapy had more advanced diseases. Interestingly, among the patients with a single liver metastasis < 50 mm in size, survival outcomes were exactly the same with or without preoperative chemotherapy (5 years: 52% vs. 57%, respectively, p = n.s.; Fig. 12.8a). Similar data were obtained for those with up to three metastases (48% and 51%, respectively, p = n.s.; Fig. 12.8b). The number of chemotherapy cycles and lines had no prognostic impact. On the contrary, survival

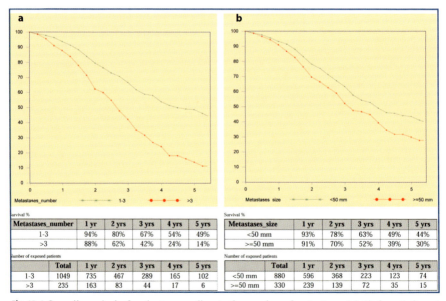

Fig. 12.6 Overall survival of patients according to the number of metastases (**a**) (1–3 vs. > 3, $p < 0.0001$) and according to the metastases size (**b**) (< 50 mm vs. ≥ 50 mm, $p = 0.003$)

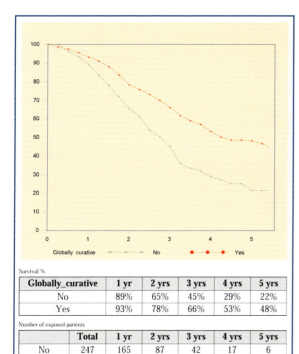

Fig. 12.7 Overall survival of patients undergoing globally curative resection (yes vs. no, $p < 0.0001$)

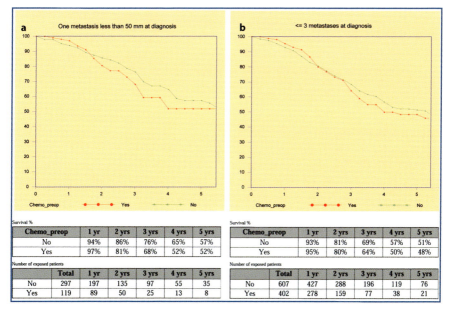

Fig. 12.8 Overall survival of patients with a single liver metastasis size < 50 mm (a) or up to 3 metastases (b) according to preoperative administration of chemotherapy (yes vs. no, p = n.s. in both cases)

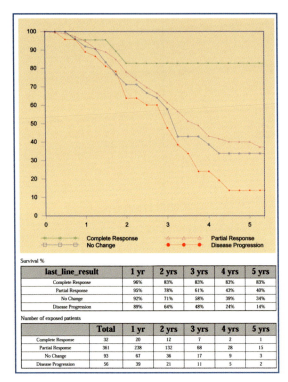

Fig. 12.9 Overall survival of patients according to the response to preoperative chemotherapy (p=0.024)

was strictly related to the response to the last chemotherapy line: the 5-year survival rate decreased from 83% after complete response to 61% after partial response, 34% after stable disease, and 14% after disease progression ($p = 0.024$; Fig. 12.9).

12.2.5
Patients with Initially Unresectable Disease

According to single-center indications, liver disease was classified as initially unresectable in 209 patients (/1348, 15.5%) who later underwent hepatic resection. The definition of unresectability was strongly associated with the number and size of the liver metastases (Fig. 12.10). The proportion of unresectable cases increased from 5.2% (33/634) in the presence of a single metastasis to 35.3% (18/51) in the presence of five metastases, to 65.4% (34/52) in the presence of ten or more metastases. Similarly, 12.2% (39/319) of the cases with lesions 30–50 mm in size and 37.1% (13/35) of those with lesions > 100 mm were classified as unresectable.

In these patients, different procedures were adopted to achieve resectability: portal vein embolization in 113, radiofrequency ablation in 95, and two-stage hepatectomy in 82. Multiple treatments were combined in 66 cases. 160 patients received conversion chemotherapy.

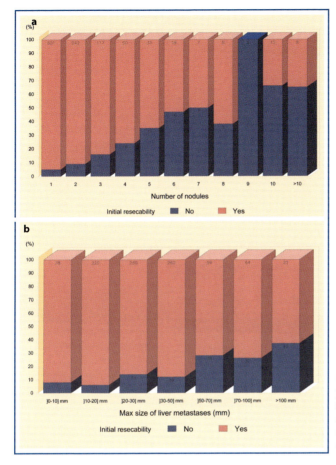

Fig. 12.10 Proportion of patients classified as unresectable at diagnosis according to the number (**a**) and the size (**b**) of liver metastases

In patients with initially unresectable disease, 3- and 5-year survival rates after resection were 47% and 20%, respectively. These results are significantly lower than those of patients with resectable disease (at 3 and 5 years 64% and 45%, respectively, $p = 0.0002$; Fig. 12.11). The 5-year survival results according to different procedures were as follows: 18% after portal vein embolization, 23% after radiofrequency ablation, and 14% after two-stage hepatectomy.

12.2.6
Comparison with the LiverMetSurvey Series

The Italian experience represents about 15% of the whole series of the LiverMetSurvey registry. Overall, the patient and tumor characteristics of this subgroup were similar to those of the whole population. Mortality was lower in the Italian group than in the whole series (1.3% vs. 3.0%), while morbidity was similar (26% vs. 28.7%). Survival rates of resected patients were the same in the two groups:

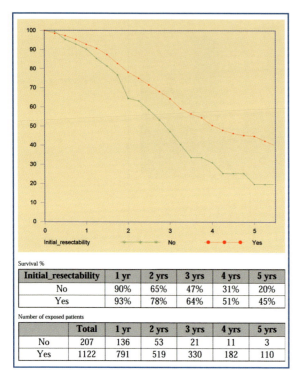

Fig. 12.11 Overall survival of patients according to the initial resectability of disease (yes vs. no, p=0.002)

at 3 and 5 years 60% and 39% in the Italian subgroup vs. 59% and 40% in the whole series (Fig. 12.12).

All prognostic factors identified in the Italian analysis were confirmed in the enlarged group; however, in the latter, additional prognostic factors were identified: age > 70 years (at 5 years 37% vs. 41%, $p = 0.0004$), primary rectal cancer (36% vs. 44%, $p < 0.0001$), synchronous presentation of the metastases (38% vs. 43%, $p = 0.002$), and number of liver metastases > 7 (21% vs. 28% for 4–7 lesions vs. 45% for 1–3 lesions, $p < 0.0001$). Considering chemotherapy, survival decreased in patients receiving multiple lines (at 5 years 40% after one line vs. 31% after two vs. 10% after three, $p < 0.0001$) and more than six cycles (37% vs. 43%, $p = 0.0002$).

12.2.7
Commentary

The Italian experience, collected in the LiverMetSurvey registry, offers a wide spectrum of surgical management of colorectal liver metastases. The results obtained thus far confirm that liver surgery is the gold standard treatment for patients with colorectal liver metastases: the 5-year survival rate is about 40% and exceeds 50% in those with a single metastasis < 50 mm. These outcomes are largely better than those achieved after explorative laparotomy (10%).

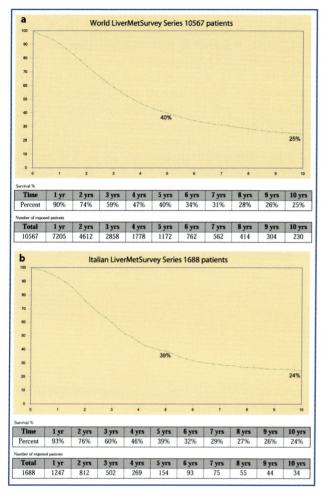

Fig. 12.12 Overall survival of patients after liver resection in the whole LiverMetSurvey series (**a**) and in the Italian series included in the LiverMetSurvey registry (**b**)

An aggressive approach to hepatic metastases can be depicted: a high proportion of patients presented with synchronous, multiple, large, or bilobar metastases. An extensive use of preoperative chemotherapy allowed the selection of good candidates for surgery and the downsizing of liver disease. About 10% of the patients underwent resection for recurrent liver metastases, achieving results similar to those obtained after the first liver resection. In the 15% of patients with initially unresectable disease, resectability was possible thanks to portal vein embolization in more than 100 cases and to two-stage hepatectomy in more than 80. Despite this aggressive approach, the mortality rate remained extremely low (1.3%) and was even lower than that in the whole LiverMetSurvey registry.

Radical resection was confirmed as the main aim of the procedure. The poor outcomes in non-radical resections suggest that surgery should be considered only if a R0 procedure can be planned. Further important prognostic factors were confirmed, such as the number and size of lesions. However the survival rates achieved in these patients clearly suggest that the presence of negative prognostic factors should not be considered a contraindication to surgery. Preoperative chemotherapy had no impact on prognosis, but this result was probably biased by the different characteristics of the patients receiving neoadjuvant treatment vs. those who did not. However, a prognostic role of response to chemotherapy was confirmed.

The role of surgery in patients with initially unresectable disease was strengthened by the observed good outcomes. Although the survival rate at 5 years was 20% and thus lower than that of patients immediately eligible for resection, it was clearly higher than the survival of patients with unresectable disease.

Finally, the treatment policy and results for colorectal liver metastases in Italy were demonstrated to be in line with those reported worldwide. Even better short-term results were obtained. In Italy, patients with colorectal metastases receive high standards of care with excellent outcomes, certainly comparable to those of other countries.

12.3
Conclusions

The present data not only confirm the literature results, but also demonstrate that large multicenter series are needed to elucidate the outcomes of surgery for colorectal liver metastases. The results of studies by tertiary referral centers have to be validated in large cohort series. Furthermore, data on the specific subgroups of patients often cannot be analyzed outside of cooperative studies because of the small number of cases. The LiverMetSurvey registry represents a well-established tool for collecting data on a large basis. The number of active centers worldwide is continuously increasing as is the number of included patients. As was done in this chapter, the survey enables the analysis of single-country results and their comparison to those of the entire database. Treatment quality and results can be checked, promoting their standardization all around the world.

Thus, all centers are invited to take part in the LiverMetSurvey database (www.livermetsurvey.org) in order to contribute to improving and standardizing the treatment of colorectal liver metastases.

Acknowledgements. The authors thank Mrs. Valérie Delvart for her contribution to statistical analysis of the data.

Subject Index

A

Adjuvant chemotherapy 60, 62, 127, 133, 143, 153-156

Adrenal metastases 139, 147, 149

B

Bevacizumab 5, 68-69, 79, 81, 83, 93-94, 114, 124-125, 128, 155, 172

C

Cetuximab 5, 78-79, 81, 83, 94, 155, 172

Colorectal
- liver metastases 2, 4, 7-10, 12-13, 15, 17, 27-30, 35, 37, 40, 43, 45, 47, 49-50, 55-60, 64-66, 68, 70-71, 85-87, 101-102, 105, 107-109, 115, 121-122, 125-126, 130, 133-134, 139-142, 148, 156, 159, 160, 162, 165, 167, 180, 182

Colorectal recurrence 140, 149

Computed tomography 10, 68, 94, 156

D

Diagnosis 1-3, 5, 12, 21-22, 75, 82, 95, 101, 107-109, 111-112, 114, 121, 139, 148, 156, 179

Disappeared metastases 83, 94, 95

E

Endoscopic stent 112-113, 115

Epidemiology 2

Extrahepatic disease 7, 18, 20, 28, 61-62, 64-65, 77, 88, 130, 139, 148-149, 156, 161-162, 171, 175-176

F

Follow-up 17, 22, 31, 47, 65, 84, 87, 95, 103, 115, 130, 134, 139-140, 144, 153, 155-156, 167, 173

Future liver remnant 29, 121-122, 124

H

Hepatic resection 4, 6, 20-21, 27, 29, 31, 37, 46-47, 49, 55, 57-58, 61, 64, 68-71, 83-87, 93-95, 103-104, 116, 125-128, 130-133, 139, 148, 154-155, 160-162, 178

Hepatectomy 28, 30, 35, 36, 41-43, 45, 49, 50, 56-58, 61, 86-88, 91, 93-96, 101, 104, 106, 116, 121, 122, 125-133, 143, 160-162, 165, 166, 173-176, 178, 179, 181

I

Indication 10, 27-31, 45, 58, 65-66, 87-89, 94, 102-104, 106-109, 122, 126, 132, 139-141, 143, 148-149, 159, 162, 178

Interstitial treatment 36, 121, 130, 132, 134

Intraoperative ultrasonography 35-36, 39, 69, 107, 166

Irinotecan 4, 29, 69, 75-83, 91, 93, 114-115, 124, 127, 155, 172

Italian experience 167, 179-180

L

Laparoscopic, Laparoscopy 35-36, 40, 45-48, 123, 132, 166

Liver
- hypertrophy 127-128
- injury 48, 90
- metastases 1-2, 4, 7-13, 15-18, 21-24, 27-30, 35, 37, 40, 43-45, 47, 49-50, 55-61, 64-68, 70-71, 76-77, 82-89, 94-95, 101-103, 105-111, 113-116, 121-122, 125-127, 130-134, 139-145, 147-148, 154-156, 159, 160, 162, 165, 167, 170, 174, 176, 178-182

LiverMetSurvey registry 166-169, 179-182

Long-term survival 27, 29, 31, 48, 61, 65, 68, 84, 159, 162

Lymph node metastases 29-30, 109, 139-142, 148-149

M

Magnetic resonance imaging 13, 95
Microwave ablation 130-133
Morbidity 47-49, 55-58, 62, 65, 84, 86-87, 91, 93, 104-106, 112, 125, 127-131, 134, 144, 159, 160, 162, 171, 179
Mortality 1, 27, 46-49, 55-57, 65, 84, 87, 91, 93-94, 104-106, 112, 125, 127-129, 131, 133-134, 144-145, 159-160, 166, 171, 179, 181

N

Natural history 4, 6, 113, 148
Neoadjuvant chemotherapy 21, 24, 28-31, 38, 45, 79, 84, 86, 88-89, 101, 103, 107-109, 116, 122, 124, 140, 143, 156

O

Oxaliplatin 5, 29, 69, 75-76, 78-80, 82-84, 90-94, 114-115, 124, 127, 153, 155, 172

P

Parenchymal 36, 42-45, 65, 91, 94, 124, 126
Pedicle clamping 35, 48-50, 104
Peritoneal carcinomatosis 29, 40, 112, 139, 143-144, 148-149,
PET 7, 17, 19-23, 94-95, 141
Portal vein
  - embolization 12, 30, 122-123, 178-179, 181
  - ligation 30, 127
  - occlusion 121-124, 129
Postoperative
  - complications 48, 55, 57, 84, 90, 122, 128
  - surveillance 7, 156
Preoperative imaging 7, 22, 40, 95, 141
Prognostic factors 28-29, 40, 48, 55, 61-62, 64, 68-71, 109, 140, 143-146, 154, 161-162, 166, 173-174, 176, 180, 182
Pulmonary metastases 111, 125, 139, 145-146, 148

R

Radiofrequency ablation 30, 47, 60, 130-132, 166, 178-179
Recurrence 3, 5, 7, 21-22, 27-28, 30-32, 35, 43, 45, 47-48, 60-61, 64, 66, 68, 70-71, 84-87, 95, 103, 107-110, 126, 129-134, 140, 147, 149, 154-156, 159, 160, 162, 166-167, 173
Re-resection 35, 156, 159, 160, 162, 173
Rescue surgery 84
Resection margin 28-32, 47

S

Scoring systems 66-68, 86
Simultaneous colorectal and liver resection 101, 104-107, 115-116
Sinusoidal dilation 89, 91-93
Staging 7-8, 17, 19, 22, 35-36, 40, 84, 107, 112, 123, 127, 140-141, 166
Steatohepatitis 89-91, 93
Steatosis 23, 50, 89-91,
Survival 4-7, 20-21, 27-29, 31-32, 37, 40, 43, 45, 47-50, 55, 58-62, 64-71, 75-76, 78, 82, 84-88, 94, 101-103, 107-110, 113, 115, 125-127, 130-134, 139-146, 148, 153-156, 159-162, 166, 172-182
Synchronous liver metastases 1-2, 87-88, 101-103, 108-110, 113-114, 116, 141, 176

T

Tumor
  - downsizing 75, 83, 94, 156
  - response 68-69, 78, 85, 87
  - staging 7, 22
Two-stage hepatectomy 30, 121, 126-131, 166, 178-179, 181

U

Ultrasound 36, 42, 55, 69, 95, 123, 132, 134, 156
Unresectable liver metastases 76, 82, 102
Up-front chemotherapy 113, 115

Printed in October 2010